THE
DEFINITIVE GUIDE
TO BURNING **FAT** AND
BUILDING **MUSCLE**

Published by CelebrityPress™, Orlando, FL
A division of The Celebrity Branding Agency®

Celebrity Branding® is a registered trademark
Printed in the United States of America.

ISBN: 9780983340423
LCCN: 2011930428

This publication is designed to provide accurate and authoritative information with regard to the subject matter covered. It is sold with the understanding that the publisher is not engaged in rendering legal, accounting, or other professional advice. If legal advice or other expert assistance is required, the services of a competent professional should be sought. The opinions expressed by the authors in this book are not endorsed by CelebrityPress™ and are the sole responsibility of the author rendering the opinion.

Most CelebrityPress™ titles are available at special quantity discounts for bulk purchases for sales promotions, premiums, fundraising, and educational use. Special versions or book excerpts can also be created to fit specific needs.

For more information, please write:

CelebrityPress™,
520 N. Orlando Ave, #2
Winter Park, FL 32789

or call 1.877.261.4930

Visit us online at www.**CelebrityPressPublishing**.com

THE DEFINITIVE GUIDE TO BURNING **FAT** AND BUILDING **MUSCLE**

TABLE OF CONTENTS:

FOREWORD

Your decision to purchase this book is probably going to turn out to be one of the smartest health and fitness decisions you've ever made.

While this book is called The Definitive Guide To Burning Fat And Building Muscle, I realize that it does not cover 'every strategy under the sun.' What it does contain, however, are the important and critical elements you need to master – in order to achieve these objectives.

As you are about to learn, what you now hold in your hands delivers the goods on the most important elements of burning fat and building muscle – and does so without getting into long treatises. One of the greatest benefits of this book is that you can get to the essence of what it takes, without reading an entire library of books. We give it all to you right here, under one cover.

This course of instruction lays the foundation for your success with the mental approach to "the game," then builds a structure of fat burning and functional muscle training on top of it. And it does so at a price that almost anyone can afford.

On the other hand, if you were to enlist my services, as well as the services of the other authors in this book, it would cost you thousands upon thousands of dollars. I say this not to boast, but to impress upon you the immense value of the information we are bringing to you.

Not only that, but please understand that the information presented in this book is RARE. You may have heard bits and pieces of it before, but never in the unique results-oriented way we'll be covering it. That's why I say you could travel all around the globe, and NOT get a tenth of the value you'll be getting here.

In fact, I dare say that just ONE of any of the lessons in this book can and probably will be worth the price of the entire manual many times over. Just take a quick look at our first chapter, if you are in doubt. In our opening lesson you'll learn how to program your mind for fat loss and muscle building in a way that guarantees results.

Now, to put this into its proper perspective, most people will tell you that success is 90 percent mental. I agree. And because I agree, I'm making sure you get a heavy prescription for your mind, up front, before we cover the physical 10 percent.

As you flip through this book you're going to learn various methods and techniques to burn fat and build muscle. No doubt you'll get excited and want to try almost everything you read, but a more practical approach would be to work with one idea at a time.

It's difficult to track results and know what's really working if you make a dozen changes all at once. A much better approach is to make one change at a time, and keep track of your results in a journal.

Perhaps you'll begin with sprint training. ...Or kettlebells. ... Or animal exercises. Whichever you choose to begin with, record what you're doing. *What gets recorded gets improved.*

So many people train mindlessly. They never test themselves to see what they're capable of achieving. Moreover, they never keep a written record of anything, so they don't know how well they're doing. If you don't know how much, how many or how fast you can do something, it's difficult to improve. On the other hand, as the saying goes: "Everyone runs faster when being timed."

This book will serve as your catalyst to greater internal as well as external strength. I wish you ten times better results than you can currently imagine.

Matt Furey

CHAPTER I

BEGIN WITH THE END IN MIND

BY MATT FUREY

Your success with this book will be predicated on following to the letter the instructions in this first lesson. Failure to heed this lesson or thinking that this is just fluff, filler or "below you" is a sure sign that you are ignorant of the most important exercise in existence. That is: putting the right thoughts into your mind.

You would not have invested in this book if you weren't influenced by the thoughts you were consciously thinking at the time. Likewise, you will not take action to give yourself the supreme levels of health and fitness you deserve, unless you begin with the end in mind. If you try to prove me wrong that would not be the part of wisdom.

So many people think that fitness success is nothing more than knowing the right movements and eating the right foods. Although that is part of the answer – the truth is you cannot get the results you want, much less stick with the right exercise or food program, unless your mind is programmed properly.

Take a look around, my friend. There are millions of people who exercise and diet and they are still fat. Why is this? The reason is because they don't understand the life-changing power that is within them. Even worse, when introduced to it, they 'flat out' reject it. They are literally afraid to take control of their thinking mechanism. Truth be told, these people fear that any attempt to harness their mind will back-fire – so instead of living the life of their dreams – they settle for whatever life hands them. They're living life by default.

This is not the way of greatness. Nor is it the way of any true student of health and fitness. You and you alone decide what it is you want in life – and you make up your mind, that 'come hell or high-water', you're going to get it.

The keys to making the transition to a consciousness that attracts success and repels failure are not difficult to learn. And they don't require a lot of time. Just follow my step-by-step instructions and you'll be on the right track in no time flat.

Let's begin with deep breathing. Why?

Three reasons, actually:

1. Breath is life. Breath is power.
2. Deep breathing calms and centers the mind.
3. Deep breathing puts you into an awakened state of awareness, **in** which you realize that you can create whatever you want in life.

Whether you are religious or not, if you take a moment to read the creation story in Genesis you'll find something interesting.

First of all, whenever God created something he pictured it in his mind first. Second, when God created the first man, he didn't come to life until God breathed life into him.

I tell you this because the whole key to making the miracles happen in your life begins the exact same way. You establish order through mentally picturing what it is that you want. Then you add power, life, vitality and energy to the mental image by breathing life into it.

The good news is, this process isn't hard to learn. Not only that, but the deep-breathing method you're about to learn will simultaneously accomplish a number of things that I just know you're going to be excited about. Instead of telling you what they are in advance, let's go over the exercise:

Here's what to do:

1. In the morning, before arising, relax with your hands at your sides.
2. Inhale deeply and fill your entire body. Imagine your body is one big lung (or balloon) – then pull the 'inhale' all the way down to your feet. Let yourself expand.
3. Once you cannot inhale further, hold for a few seconds, then begin to exhale.
4. During the 'exhale' squeeze your abdominals as if you're wringing water from a towel. Squeeze them from the top to bottom.
5. As you squeeze, exhale slowly making a "sssss" sound. Continue making this sound and squeezing until your inhale is completely finished. Leave nothing in the lungs. Get everything out.
6. Also, while exhaling and squeezing your abdominals, it is a healthy practice for you to follow what many

great Indian and Chinese *chi kung* practitioners teach, i.e. – to contract and pull up on your perineum. This will not only improve your overall energy – but will greatly improve your sex life.

7. Do this deep breathing exercise 10 times in the morning before getting out of bed. You are then welcome to get up, stand before an open window and do more of the same. You can also do this exercise anytime throughout the day, especially when you need to "energize" or rid yourself of mental stress.

Now that you've read over these instructions, take a few minutes and do this breathing technique 10 times. In order to get you fired up about it even more, and just in case you missed the benefits in the steps outlined above, here are some of the many benefits of this type of breathing:

• Increases mental alertness and clarity
• Increases creativity and mental power
• Rids your body and mind of negative stress
• Increases energy
• Tightens, tones and strengthens the abdominals
• Improves digestion and elimination
• Cleans the lungs of stale energy
• Helps you to relax
• Improves overall power due to strengthening of core muscles
• Improves functioning of sexual organs

Enough said. Now do your 10 repetitions and get a feel for how powerful this technique actually is.

****

Okay, good. Once you've finished your set of 10 deep breaths, you should feel that you have moved into a different vibration. Put simply, you should feel good all over.

And that good feeling is the KEY to success in life, especially when you know how to harness it and combine it with other mental programming techniques.

The bottom line is that we don't just become what we think about – as the sages have said. We become what we think about with "deep emotion." To merely think a thought doesn't give it a lot of power. But to think a thought backed by an abundance of enthusiasm and positive emotion – well, let me just say "look out world." Because here you come.

Understand that we think in pictures. That is crucial to achieve whatever your aims are.

For example, think of your home. What comes to mind? A mental picture, right?

Now think of your car; your wardrobe; your library, your television; your favorite restaurant. And so on. What did you see? One picture right after the other, correct?

Well, now form a mental picture of the type of physique you want to have. Do you want to get big and huge? Or do you want to get lean and ripped? Either desire can be met with this program. I have proven it.

As you know, although Gama was only 5' 7" tall, he hit a bodyweight of 260 pounds. Taking a page from his book, and doing so to prove that "yes" you can get bigger and stronger with bodyweight exercises, I went on a weight-gain program with the training and dietary regimen outlined in this course. And guess what? I continued to grow and get stronger. And my weight reached an all-time high of 238 pounds.

This is no different than weight training in that some people train with weights to get HUGE and others do so to get lean. So we know it can be done. But most people erroneously believe that you get big from the exercise itself. You don't. You can do all the classic power lifts and Olympic lifts and NOT gain weight. It's done all the time.

So what then, is the key to gaining or losing weight with an exercise program? Quite simply, the key is your intention. What is it that you want? Tell your muscles what you want them to do with the exercises and they will obey.

Your flesh has an intelligence and it simply sits back and waits for you to give it orders. Once the orders are given, every cell in your body goes to work to shape your body the way you want it.

We know that people who are sick can make themselves well by the thoughts they think. We also know that perfectly healthy people can make themselves sick by thinking negatively. It happens every day in every city in the world.

Yet, we miss the boat and think this doesn't apply to fitness. It does.

Ed Baran, whom you'll see in this book, used the same training regimen I follow, albeit a different diet, to get ripped and lean. He went from a bodyweight of 215 pounds to 190. How did he do this?

Well, first and foremost, by WANTING to do so. Second, by thinking about his goal all the time, And third, by holding this image in mind while he trained. It's as simple as that.

The unrevealed "trick" to all of this, though, is not just picturing what you want – but picturing it with conviction. Put some white-heat behind your desire and you cannot help but go in the direction of what you want. This we know to be a Universal LAW. Put it to use and the world is your oyster.

Now, how do you add positive emotion to your goal? Very simple.

While inhaling and energizing your entire being, form a mental picture of your desire. Now, quite literally, surround the mental image (your goal) with breath. Instead of focusing on squeezing your abdominals, however – which you did through the formation of a mental picture and a verbal command (self-talk), you squeeze (add emotion) to the mental image.

Now, after you've completed your inhale, begin your exhale. But instead of merely letting off steam, surround your mental image with this energy. Literally exhale right into the image, surrounding it with your power.

Understand that there is a reason why the Taoists of China always begin their martial arts practice with deep breathing exercises. The same is done before anything creative is attempted. Whether painting, drawing, writing or singing – you start with breath.

Now, once again, think back to the story of creation as told in Genesis. Remember the key I mentioned earlier?

God breathed life into Adam.

Whether you believe the Biblical story of creation or not is NOT my point. My point is that the practice described in Genesis is exactly what you want to use in your own life. Always remember that you are not just a MAN (or Woman) – you are a being with the same creative God-like ability written about in Genesis. After all, if man was made in the image and likeness of God – and God is a creator – then it makes sense that man is also a creator – and is happiest and most God-like when he is creating.

This is why goals are so important. We are happiest when we are creating. We are less than happy, if not just plain miserable, when we aren't. So form a goal and add life to it through your deep breathing practice. Begin and end every workout with deep breathing. Begin and end each day with deep breathing. Never begin a creative endeavor of any sort without taking a few minutes to do some deep breathing.

Will it change your results? Big time!

Now, let me close this first lesson by having you do a couple written exercises that are vitally important. Do NOT overlook these. If you want to soar like an eagle, hark unto me and pay attention.

Many people, when asked to define what it is they want in life literally draw a blank. They can't think clearly about what they want because their mind has been so preoccupied with what they DON'T want for so long, that it appears that there is nothing else.

Never forget that we become what we habitually think about with deep emotion. And so, if you can't even think of what you want because you've got too much invested in what you don't want – guess what you're creating? That's right. More of what you DON'T want.

Well, my friend, there is a way out of that 'hell-hole.' So, Before you make a list of what you want, let's make a list of what you don't want.

Take out a pen and get ready to fill out the following page with...

Things I Don't Want To Do or Have No Mo'

Now, beneath this headline start rattling them off. List everything that comes to mind. For example...

I don't want to be fat.
I don't want to be weak.
I don't want anymore back pain.
I don't want these headaches.
I don't want to wear clothes made for an elephant.
I don't want women to turn me down.
I don't want to be afraid to workout in public.

And so on.

Get the idea. It's not hard. Just move your pen across the paper and write whatever comes to mind. Do it Now!

Please. Do it. Don't move on until you've done this. Put your pen on the next page and fill it with things you don't want to do anymore or that you want to eliminate from your life.

Things I Don't Want To Do or Have No Mo'

_____

_____

_____

_____

_____

_____

_____

_____

_____

_____

_____

_____

_____

_____

_____

_____

_____

_____

_____

_____

_____

Alrighty, then. After you're done writing the list of things you don't want – your mind will be clearer than ever before. This means that you're finally ready to make a list of what you DO want.

Bear in mind that you can write anything on this list that you want. It doesn't have to be fitness related. But a few of the items should be fitness oriented because that's the subject you're studying here.

So here's what you do. On the following page under the headline… **Things I Want To Create In My Life – you'll want to write out 10 things you want to achieve within the next 12 months.**

For example, your list might be something like this:

> I want to be able to do 500 straight Hindu squats.
> I want to weigh 170 pounds and have a 32-inch waist.
> I want to fit into the clothes I wore three years ago.
> I want to own a brand new Corvette.
> I want to double my current income.
> I want to attract the perfect mate into my life.
> I want to earn $50,000 in my new business.

Okay, got the idea? Super. Then take a few minutes and jot down the top 10 goals you want to achieve over the next 12 months. Do it NOW!

Things I Want To Create in My Life

_____

_____

_____

_____

_____

_____

_____

_____

_____

_____

_____

_____

_____

_____

_____

_____

_____

_____

_____

_____

_____

Good job!

Now that you have your 10 goals written out, you can always go back to them later on and add more details. The more vivid the details, the better the result. The key, however, is getting started and putting something on paper.

CHOOSING ONE GOAL

The next thing to do after you made the two lists is to select one goal that you want to focus on over the next month. Choose something that you can achieve in under 30 days; even in as little as seven days. If you don't have a goal that is short-term, then take a few moments and come up with one.

The purpose of having a short-term goal is to build confidence quickly. Once you know you can focus on a goal and make it happen – then your creative power grows by leaps and bounds, and you tackle and accomplish bigger and bigger tasks at faster and faster speeds.

Once you have selected the one goal you are going to focus on – write it on a 3x5 card (or the goal card I gave you with this program) and give it a deadline for accomplishment. For example, you might write something like the following:

> ***"By December 31, I can and I will do***
> ***100 straight Hindu pushups."***

Or something to that effect.

Now, each day when you get up, focus on this goal. Picture yourself having already accomplished it. And while you picture it, add emotion to it. Add the breath of life to the image. Feel the enthusiasm. Feel the deep, positive emotion.

Carry the 3x5 card with you everywhere you go. Keep it in

your front pants pocket. Or put it in your wallet. Take it out each day and read it several times with DEEP CONVICTION.

Then, when you do your workout – notice how much more focused you are. Notice how much harder you train.

Most importantly, notice how fast you improve.

While you train, tell yourself, "I Can. I Will. I Can. I Will."

Then add the ending to it, "I can and I will do 100 straight Hindu pushups by December 31."

What I have just taught you is the MASTER KEY to achieving anything you want in life. Without it you can achieve very little.

To me, this first lesson is the most important of them all. Anyone can teach you exercises. Anyone can teach you a diet to follow. But the whole key to making any of it work lies inside of YOU.

In case you're wondering whether or not I follow the advice I've given you here, let me just say the following:

While in college I had a 3x5 card with a goal written on it. I carried it with me everywhere. It predicted that I would become a national champion. And guess what? I became one.

Today, some 18 years after that goal became an accomplished fact, I still use 3x5 cards all the time. It's either in my pocket or upon my desk. Each time a goal is achieved the 3x5 card is replaced with a new one, giving me a new target to shoot for.

This focusing technique has helped me accomplish whatever I set my mind on.

But does it work for someone else? It sure does. Last August I received the following proof from an overjoyed customer who used the technique. This is what he had to say:

> *Matt,*
>
> *Wanted* to *get this* to ya sooner, *but been working* a *ton. Man I* owe *you BIG time, Matt. I've purchased* a *lot of* your *products in the past (Combat Conditioning, Combat Abs, Power Wheel, etc.), but it was the* focus *of your newsletter in July that really produced results!!*
>
> *On July 14, 2002, I ran the Utica Boilermaker 15K* (9.3 *miles) road race. Now I've* run *this race since* 1986 *with* my *best time being* 72 *minutes and some change. I've always wanted* to *get below* 70 *minutes, but never came close.*
>
> *Well,* I *read your article about goals (about* 6 *days before the race) and wrote out* my *goal time* (69:54) my *splits and some positive thoughts.* I *would look* at *it many, many times each day. I headed* out at *the gun and felt great, with* no *negative thoughts* or *aches* or *pains and finished in* 69: 06!!! *(at* 45 *years old).*
>
> *Matt, thanks again from the bottom of* my *heart. You RULE!!!!*
>
> *Marty J.*
> *New Hartford,* NY
> *(#1278 out of 10,000 finishers)*

Yes, you can take charge of your life. Marty is proof of that. He not only beat his previous best time in that race – he <u>shattered</u> it. Just by focusing on the target and adding passion to it, he knocked three minutes off his time.

Need I say more?

Follow the suggestions in this opening lesson, and you'll be the master of your body.

[This chapter comes from Lesson One in my Gama Fitness course, available in written and DVD form at Gama-Fitness.com]

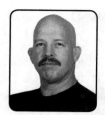

ABOUT MATT

Matt Furey was born in a small town in Iowa, named Carroll.

At eight years of age he began competing in swimming and wrestling and through dedicated practice became a champion in both. In 1981, Matt Furey was the state runner-up in the Class 3A Iowa High School State Wrestling Championships at 167-pounds. He attended The University of Iowa from 1981-1984, where he wrestled for Olympic Gold medalist, Dan Gable, and was a member of three national championship teams.

In the fall of 1984, in order to help rebuild a doormat wrestling program, Furey transferred to Edinboro University of Pennsylvania, and in 1985 he won the NCAA II national title at 167-pounds, defeating two-time California state champion, Howard Lawson, in the finals. While at Edinboro he was coached by Mike DeAnna and two-time Olympic Gold Medalist Bruce Baumgartner.

In February of 1987, Furey opened a personal training business for wrestlers and fitness enthusiasts. Most of the high school wrestlers he trained went on to wrestle in college.

Furey began studying various martial arts in 1990 and immediately saw the physical, mental and philosophical links these arts had with wrestling. This lead to the publication of his first book and videos in 1996, entitled, *The Martial Art of Wrestling*.

Also in 1996, Furey began competing in the ancient Chinese grappling art of Shuai-Chiao, the oldest style of kung fu. Furey's teacher, Dr. Daniel Weng, a national champion from Taiwan, and a ninth-degree black belt, guided Furey to three national titles.

During Christmas of 1997, Dr. Weng brought two U.S. teams to Beijing, China, to compete in the world championships. In Beijing, Furey won the gold medal at 90 KG (198-pounds), and was the only non-Chinese to win a title. In addition, Furey's world title was historic because it marked the first time that an American had won a gold medal in any world kung fu competition held in China.

In the spring of 1998, Furey was inducted into the Edinboro University of Pennslyvania Athletic Hall of Fame.

In 1999, Furey traveled to Tampa, Florida to train under the legendary Karl Gotch. Several months later Furey moved his family from California to Tampa, Florida, so he could train with Gotch full-time. Gotch taught Furey a treasure trove of knowledge on conditioning as well as the real professional style of wrestling, known as catch-as-catch-can (catch wrestling).

Furey's unique experience as a Chinese kung fu and wrestling champion, earned him covers for *Grappling, Inside Kung Fu, Karate Illustrated, Gladiator* and *Martial Arts Illustrated*.

In 2002, *Grappling* magazine dubbed Furey, "The King of Catch Wrestling" – and in the book *Grappling Masters*, Furey is one of 22 elite world class grapplers who are interviewed and featured.

In 2010, *Inside Kung Fu* named Furey as their *Hall of Fame Writer of the Year*.

Furey is also the author of the international best-selling **Combat Conditioning**, as well as **Combat Abs**, *The Unbeatable Man*, *101 Ways to Magnetize Money, The Fastest Way Humanly Possible to Burn Fat*, **Combat Stretching**, **Gama Fitness** and **Magnetic Mind Power**.

As President of *The Psycho-Cybernetics Foundation*, Furey is dedicated to spreading the teachings of Dr. Maxwell Maltz, author of the 30-million copy best-seller, *Psycho-Cybernetics*.

Along with his wife and two children, Furey resides in Tampa, Florida and Hainan Island, China.

CHAPTER 2

BACK PAIN: GETTING A BREAK FROM THE ACHE

BY DR. MERICK ABRAJANO, D.C.

When it comes to maintaining a reasonable level of physical fitness – or even just going about your everyday life – back pain can really cramp your style. It's something I understand firsthand, because I too was briefly a victim of excruciating back pain.

It happened back when I was an accounting major in college with no intention of becoming a chiropractor. As it turns out, fate had other ideas. I was outside, enjoying a ride on my 10 speed in a cycling class at California State University, Long Beach, when I took an unexpected detour into a ditch. It wasn't a happy landing.

That two-wheel disaster left me with severe back pain, nothing you want to deal with as a college student (or at any other time in your life, for that matter). I went to my HMO doctor and his solution was to prescribe pain pills for me. They didn't really help. I was uncomfortable and I didn't feel up to much physical activity.

This went on for several months – more pills, more pain, no relief. I was at a loss as to how I could resolve this ongoing and debilitating problem, when finally, someone suggested I go see a chiropractor. Having nothing left to lose, except a few dollars for the visit, I decided I would check him out.

And in my first session, he made the pain go away.

This was a like a miracle to me. I couldn't imagine that someone could instantly solve what was rapidly starting to appear to me to be a problem without a solution.

After that semester, I transferred all my credits and pursued a career in chiropractic medicine. Oh, and I had to make a few other alterations in my personal appearance as well. At the time I was the drummer for a heavy metal band named "Heretic," so my hairstyle was a little less than…professional. And the first thing I was told when applying for chiropractic school was to chop off my long, flowing mane of Metallica-like hair.

I don't think the hair would have made me less of a chiropractor. But I undoubtedly scare fewer patients with my current look! I'm sure it's responsible for me running a successful practice for 16 years, as well as being proud to serve as the team doctor for the 2004 Olympic Decathlon team.

BACK PAIN: FACTS AND FIGURES

Back pain is an incredibly common problem in America. At

any given time, 31 million Americans experience low-back pain, according to the American Chiropractic Association (ACA). As a matter of fact, experts estimate that as many as 80% of the entire population will experience a back problem at some point in our lives. I'm sure many of you reading this chapter either have had back problems or know someone who has.

Back pain is also a large drain on our productivity. It's one of the most widespread reasons for missing work, as well as being the second most common cause of doctor visits (upper-respiratory infections is number one). Not only that, but Americans spend over $50 billion every year seeking back pain remedies – and those are just the costs we can easily identify.

Why is back pain so common?

Well, the back itself is a complex structure of muscles, bones, joints and ligaments – all of which are subject to damage. Ligaments can sprain, muscles can strain, disks can rupture and joints can be irritated, all of which can lead to back pain. It doesn't take incredible acrobatics or feats of sport to in-stigate a painful back injury – or riding a bicycle in a ditch, for that matter. It can often be an incredible simple everyday motion, such as bending over to pick up your shoes, or turn-ing your body a certain way. Professional athletes have suf-fered major back injuries not because of what they've done on the field, but because of performing what would seem to be a normal task for any of us.

In addition, back pain can happen as a result of indirect causes as well – such as arthritis, poor posture, obesity and even stress, not to mention other diseases of internal organs such as kidney stones, kidney infections, blood clots or bone loss.

Chiropractic medicine has been shown to be one of the most effective methods to relieve back pain in the world. Established in 1890, it is now the third largest health industry, behind only medicine and dentistry.

Although chiropractic medicine has been controversial in the past, it is now well-established and even recommended by the U.S. government. After an extensive study of all currently available care for low back problems, the U.S. Agency for Health Care Policy and Research recommended chiropractic treatment as the only safe and effective, drugless form of initial professional treatment for acute low back problems in adults.

WHY SURGERY IS USUALLY NOT THE BEST SOLUTION

As I mentioned earlier, chiropractic medicine has been a bit controversial in the past. The American Medical Association boycotted chiropractors until 1987, when they lost an antitrust case; it now is largely accepted by both medical doctors as well as health insurance plans.

I found from my own experience, which I discussed earlier in this chapter, that sometimes mainstream medicine just doesn't know how to handle back pain and back injuries. To tell you the truth, my practice, The Southland Spine Center in Torrance, California, has helped many people who just couldn't find any solutions from their usual doctors.

Our specialty is those that have found no relief from their ongoing chronic back pain through any other channel. They've been through injuries, they've had pain management shots, and their agony just doesn't stop. As a matter of fact, their doctors have argued that the only thing that can help most of them is back surgery.

That's when they usually come to us – because they don't want to deal with the pain, expense and the post-rehabilitation period that accompanies back surgery. More importantly, there's the fact that there's a very good chance that *it simply won't work.*

Doctors themselves will tell you that the failure rate for back surgery is 51%. There's even a term for this negative outcome – Failed Back Surgery Syndrome (FBSS) – which can leave the patient with a greater degree of chronic back pain than he or she had before the surgery. Even though there is no guarantee back surgery will work, the popularity of the procedure continues to skyrocket – from 122,000 operations in 2001 to over 500,000 in 2006, with a price tag in the billions of dollars.

On the other hand, we have been able to help 91% of all the patients we see that have had back surgery recommended as their only viable option for relief.

HOW WE HELP

We treat many of these patients who are seeking to avoid surgery with our NSSD Therapy. Utilizing ultrasound and interferential therapies, our techniques create a negative pressure in the lumbar spine that pulls back a patient's bulging discs, taking the strain off the nerves which is causing the back pain.

The advantages to nonsurgical spinal decompression are many, including:

- It is non-invasive
- It is effective and safe
- It has none of the risks associated with drugs and/or anesthesia

- Resolution of symptoms is long-lasting.

Once the patient's pain is under control, we start them on our ATM®2 exercise machines – ATM stands for Active Therapy Movement. This is a relatively new device in the field of physical therapy whose primary purpose is to restore *pain-free* range of motion (ROM) in the spine, whether it is the low back, mid-back or neck. ATM is a process whereby isometric exercise of the spine in a stabilized, pain-free position is utilized to regain the motion of the spine apart from pain.

The ATM®2 helps strengthen the multifidus muscles, which are the small ones next to the spine that are never rehabilitated. We tackle whichever motion causes the patient pain by locking in their spine and pelvis using an interlocking belt system.

We then use another machine, called a Med-X Extension, to strengthen the posterior lumbar spinal muscles in the back of the spine. Later on we use a Med-X Flexion machine, to strengthen the muscles in front of the spine.

Finally, when the patient is ready to move on to the next step, we use yet another large machine called a Med-X Rotation to strengthen the muscles along the sides of the spine. In conjunction with the work on the machines in our offices, we also give our patients a customized, specific exercise and stretching program that they can do at home.

With strengthened spine muscles, the vast majority of our patients can finally move beyond their back pain and get on with their lives.

Are you a candidate for our nonsurgical spinal decompression treatment? Only a consultation with us can tell, but here are a few questions that you should ask yourself:

- Are you dependant on daily medications?
- Are your everyday activities limited by back pain?
- Have you had repeated spinal injections or epidurals with no relief?
- Are you considering spinal surgery, or has your doctor recommended it – and are you confused about that choice?
- Have you tried chiropractic or physical therapy with no success?
- Have you missed a lot of work, or been out of work, due to pain?

If "yes" is the answer to any of the above questions, this might be the right treatment path for you to follow.

Not everyone is the right fit for general chiro care. That chronic low back and neck pain, along with radiating arm and leg pain that's caused by protruding or herniated disc, are better resolved with a non surgical medical technology known as NSSD Therapy. This is what I utilize in my clinic due to the high risk and poor outcomes often associated with heavy duty narcotic pain meds, epidural steroid injections and risky surgical procedures.

AVOIDING BACK PAIN

Fortunately, most of us don't have this kind of severe pain – but we all tend to get the occasional backache from what we do in our normal lives. There are ways to minimize this kind of discomfort, so here are some tips on how to prevent back pain from ruining your day:

- Maintain a healthy diet and weight.
- Remain active—under the supervision of your doctor of chiropractic.
- Avoid prolonged inactivity or bed rest.

- Warm up or stretch before you exercise or do any other physical activities, such as gardening.
- Maintain proper posture.
- Wear comfortable, low-heeled shoes.
- Sleep on a mattress of medium firmness to minimize any curve in your spine.
- Lift with your knees, keep the object close to your body, and do not twist when lifting.
- Stop smoking. Smoking impairs blood flow, resulting in oxygen and nutrient deprivation to spinal tissues (as a matter of fact, smokers have the most complications following back surgery).
- Work with your doctor of chiropractic to ensure that your computer workstation is ergonomically correct.

For most of us, back pain is an occasional inconvenience that we have to bite our lip and get through until its better. For others, however, chronic back pain can deeply affect their quality of life, until it affects their job performance, their personal relationships and their very ability to enjoy life.

Going beyond the usual medical treatments to what chiropractic medicine has to offer, can help many of those back pain victims avoid expensive back surgery – that may not even solve the problem.

We all want to enjoy physical health and physical fitness to fully appreciate our lives. When it comes to back pain, getting "a break from the ache" allows us all to do just that.

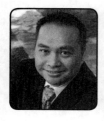

ABOUT MERICK

Dr. Merick Abrajano, D.C. is the Clinic Director of Southland Spine Center in the Torrance, CA area. He has been in practice for 17 years and is a local authority and patient advocate for back and disc pain sufferers.

Dr. Abrajano has revealed that what many think about back pain, disc pain, sciatica, unresolved back pain, leg and hip pain, bulging and slipped discs may in fact be completely WRONG! And while his opinions are not shared by everyone in the back and disc pain field, ...this doctor's perspective is hard to ignore, and he appears to have an army of smiling happy patients (FORMER back and disc pain sufferers), ready to vouch for him and his spine center.

In 2004, he was team doctor for the Olympic Decathlon Team, and has treated many elite athletes and sports stars. He currently resides in Palos Verdes, California with his wife and three children.

To learn more about Dr. Merick Abrajano, and how you can receive a free special report and other invaluable information from one of the country's leading experts, visit www.TorranceBackPainDoctor.com or call Toll-Free 1-800-298-1338.

Contact info:

drmerick@southlandspinecenter.com
www.southlandspinecenter.com

CHAPTER 3

GOLFING YOUR WAY TO BETTER HEALTH

BY CHIPPER JIMMY (JIM BRADLEY)

If you are searching for an exercise activity, please don't overlook golf. There are a variety of golfing experiences available that can give you anything from a very mild exercise experience to a brisk walk of 6 to 8 miles. Whether you are aged, suffering from a physical challenge of some sort, or currently fairly fit, you can probably find a golfing exercise experience that is appropriate for you.

Although golf won't turn you into a Green Beret, studies have shown that even mild exercise is beneficial, and for many, mild exercise is all they can safely handle, now.

For those looking for something more strenuous, playing golf (walking, not riding in a motorized cart) at full-length courses, will provide more than the recommended 150 minutes of medium level activity per week that many fitness organizations recommend.

Even if you are very badly out of shape, and can't physically make a full golf swing, there is a way for you to incorporate golf into your fitness regime. The key thing to remember is that generally speaking, when it comes to exercise, although more is usually better, doing anything is better than doing nothing.

I believe that playing golf is the perfect exercise for modern people, because, ironically, it's "caveman" exercise. Our bodies have not changed much from caveman days. I believe that the human body, probably like the bodies of most other animals, is made to do a lot a walking. If you look at the activities of the few people on the planet who still live primitive lifestyles, you'll see that they spend a lot of time walking. They walk for several hours searching for game, and searching for other edible things to eat. Just like cavemen did.

As primitive foragers search for food, they walk for long distances, pausing for short intervals whenever they find a few berries, or a few seeds. Compare this to modern man, who takes long breaks in the snack foods section of a super-market before taking a short walk to the baked goods section. Primitive people find their food scattered over a wide area, and so they walk. Once in a while they exert themselves to throw a bola at a bird, or a spear at a monkey.

Taking relatively long walks between short pauses to make a golf shot is like being a modern day caveman. You may walk more or less continuously for 4 or 5 hours, taking frequent pauses to make a shot. (Hopefully not TOO frequently, as the goal, after all, is to take as few shots as possible!)

Now, of course, we ARE talking about walking the course.

Unless you get a surprise invitation to play Augusta and they insist on your using a cart, you should be walking when you golf. Why pass up a great opportunity for the gentle, but continuous exercise your body was designed for?

Here is the golf "ladder," with each rung giving you a little more of a work out.

If you are badly out of shape, or can't make a full golf shot because of a physical limitation, you could find a putting golf course and play there. These courses have holes that are from 30 to 100 yards long and you play them with only a ball and a putter. All shots are putts. You could even just play a couple holes and build up, if you needed to. In golf, you can play yourself into shape. Try doing that in rugby!

Putting courses are fun, good putting practice, and are a great way for the aged or infirm to get outdoors, be active within their limitations, and enjoy some of the masochistic fun of chasing that little white ball that golfers on longer courses have.

Perhaps the next rung on the golf ladder – pitch-and-putt courses – would be appropriate for your first golf experiences. These are very short courses where you do make some full swings, although the holes may be as short as 65 yards or so.

If you play a pitch-and-putt course, you may only walk a mile. This may enough for seniors and those who are, for various reasons, not able to do more. A pitch-and-putt course will get these people out in the fresh air, and walking on natural surfaces in gently challenging conditions. And enjoying some of the masochistic fun...

If you are in between being able to play a putting only course and a whole pitch-and-putt, you could always just play a few holes of the pitch and putt, or even just one hole to start, and build up, adding holes as you gain stamina.

From pitch and putt courses, you can graduate to the next rung up the golf ladder – the so-called "executive" style courses. These are courses that are longer than pitch-and-putts, but still quite a bit shorter than full-length courses. These courses usually are from 2,500 to 3,500 yards, and would make a pleasant workout for people adding to their fitness levels. If you felt that you couldn't handle walking the full course, you would have the option to only play 9 holes.

The final rung up the golf ladder is the "full length course" rung. Here you will be playing courses that usually have 10 par 4 holes, 4 par 3 holes, and 4 par 5 holes. Most full-length courses that amateurs play are between 5,500 and 7,000 yards long. That's right around 4 miles. But unless you're a PGA tour player, I'm guessing that you're going to be walking a little to the left after this shot, and a little to the right, maybe, after the next. You know – military golf! Left, right, left, right! That means that you'll probably be walking from 6 to 8 miles every time you play 18 holes. That's a good workout!

Most courses have some elevation changes, and hazards (I mean… "challenges!") that you might have to climb into and out of. These add to the workout you'll be receiving from your "stroll." On full-length courses, you could again start out by playing just 9 holes instead of the entire 18 holes.

Here's a fun way to play all 18 holes of a full-length course and walk only 9 holes. Find a buddy, a date, or a spouse who shares your interest in golf and fitness, and golf with him/her. Rent a cart, but take turns walking every other hole. One rides, one walks, switch. If you are going to golf and walk, as

I suggest you do, make sure that you get either a very good carry bag with very good shoulder straps to making carrying clubs convenient and safe for your back, or an excellent pull or push cart for your clubs.

Pull or push carts can be obtained that fold up conveniently for transporting in your car. They are worth their weight in gold. Make sure you get one with large diameter wheels and wheels that are wide, as well. That will make traversing the sometimes uneven terrain of the course much easier. (You might have to pull or push your cart through a bit of rough. I know that YOU wouldn't ever hit your shot there, but a seagull or a coyote might grab your perfectly struck ball from its position in the exact middle of the fairway and drop it in the fescue!)

Make sure that your golf shoes are in good condition. You don't want sore feet and blisters. If you need orthotics, get them. If your feet are tired at the end of a round, visit your podiatrist (foot doctor). Wear socks that wick away moisture, and possibly sock liners, to prevent blisters.

***A note on style: please, guys, just for me, don't let the only thing white in your attire be your socks!*

As before starting any exercise program, consult a physician before starting a golfing exercise program, and okay it with him or her. A good reason to consult your doctor now about exercise is that you may be wrongly assuming, if you have some health concerns, that you shouldn't be exercising, when in fact your doctor WANTS you to get active, and is eager to advise you on how to begin.

Tell your physician about any conditions that you know about that may make him or her suggest limits to your activity. For instance, if you are pregnant, there may be precautions your doctor will want you to take. If you have arthritis, or other joint problems, your doctor may suggest that you forego golf, or take precautions to protect yourself. He or she may suggest special padded grips that are meant for arthritic golfers, and graphite shafts that may absorb more shock at impact than do regular shafts.

He or she may suggest placing your ball on a tee for every shot, to lesson impact stress. Yes, that's illegal on the PGA tour, but you're golfing for fun and exercise, not to win the U.S. Open, right?

A word of caution now on the dangers of golfing off mats. Some ranges, some pitch-and-putts, and some executive length courses have mats that you must tee off from. My mother, at the tender age of 75, decided to take up golf. She proceeded to hit down onto an unforgiving mat in an attempt to hit a tee shot, and tore her right upper arm muscle so badly that surgery wasn't even an option.

If you have to hit off mats, don't! Just make a little putting like stroke to get the ball 4 or 5 yards off the mat, and then commence golfing from there. You don't have to count that first stroke, but you did begin from the mat, just like the management wanted you to!

When the doctor gives you the green light to go, go gradually. If you're badly out of shape, a walk of only 5 minutes may be enough for the first day. Take a while to build up endurance. You can start by playing one hole of a putting only course, and build up from there.

It's all about getting out and doing SOMETHING, which, according to the British Heart Foundation, is better than doing nothing. If you're training to be a Navy Seal, go ahead and run around 'full tilt' with your buddies, carrying a telephone pole over your heads. Otherwise, do a reasonable amount of something that you enjoy enough to keep doing.

Think about your diet while you're golfing, as well as at other times. Your body will need the right kind of energy. Forget about the hotdog, chips and beer halfway through your round. Most recent nutritional advice is trending towards favoring a whole food, plant-based diet. I say, "Hey, that's a cave-man diet! Just right for our cave-man bodies."

Krok may have been a mighty hunter, but he ate mostly seeds, fruit, and nuts. When he did knock over the occasional mastodon, it was party time and instant weekend. But after gorging his great belly with chops, he didn't go golfing. He lay down, like a lion after feeding, and went to sleep.

After the front nine, try a banana, or an almond butter sandwich made with whole grain bread. These complex carbohydrates will give you the slow but steady release of energy that your body needs while being active. Don't give it sugar – that's like putting drag-racing car fuel into a Honda Civic. Stay hydrated. Don't wait until you feel thirsty to start drinking. Drink proactively, and avoid alcohol while golfing. Alcohol may make you smarter, funnier, sexier, and better looking, (yeah, right!)... but it will de-hydrate you.

Avoid so-called "sports drinks" which contain a lot of sugar. Talk to your naturopath or health foods store advisor about the kind of fluids you should be drinking while exercising outdoors, in the heat. They may recommend an alkalizing drink of some sort. Some researchers feel that an acidic body is more prone to illness and fatigue. Don't forget to take proper skincare precautions, as you will be out in the sun. Protect your eyes, too, from too much sun, by wearing good quality sunglasses.

Taking these precautions, and building up your golfing exercise program gradually can only benefit you – especially if you are sedentary now. Let yourself be beguiled by the world's hardest, but most enthralling game. Your overall health may improve, and your waistline may shrink while you hone your swearing skills!

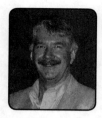

ABOUT JIM

Jim Bradley is the Internet's foremost authority on overcoming frustration while golfing.

Introduced to golf by a low-handicap girl-friend, Jim soon discovered golfing frustration, as he sought to quickly match her on-course achievements.

Frustrated golfers of the world, Jim feels your pain! In the past he did it all: threw clubs, 'busted' clubs, and attacked golf bags. ...And invented new swearing phrases to match almost any situation.

Jim's golf game was turning violent – he was beating up on himself! After watching the movie "Happy Gilmour," Jim decided he didn't want to be an angry golfer anymore, and set out to learn to golf without frustration.

His efforts led to the development of his Frustration Free Golf program, which comes in various forms, from the full program to the "Emergency program."

And it's all available at www.frustrationfreegolf.com

Originally from Lethbridge, Alberta, Canada, Jim now lives in Vancouver, B.C., Canada. He is a pilot for an international airline and has chased the little white ball on several continents.

As well as golfing, Jim shoots clay pigeons, and is a former provincial champion. He is also interested in most other facets of fitness and health.

CHAPTER 4

'CLIMB THE MOUNTAIN' WITH KETTLEBELLS

BY VICTOR CRAWFORD

"Not a single sport develops our muscular strength and bodies as well as Kettlebell athletics."

~ Russian Magazine *Hercules*-1913

THE KETTLEBELL PHENOMENON

Undoubtedly you have heard of them. You've probably even seen them somewhere and wondered to yourself, "What is that menacing looking thing?" You may have even placed wagers with your friends about what they are. If you haven't heard of them, you haven't been paying attention because they are sweeping our industry like a forest fire. They have been referred to as "cowbells," "kettle balls," and the like. But the cannonballs with a handle that you swing with one or both hands over in the corner of the gym are called Kettlebells, and if used appropriately, they will whip your butt into shape fast. They come in different sizes and weights, so they are very versatile depending on a particular person's goals and objectives.

THE WORD ON THE STREET

So, besides looking good and feeling good, why on earth would you or should you use kettlebells as your fitness machine of choice? Well, there are many reasons, which I will elaborate on, in a bit. But first I would like to explain further why *I* began to use them, and what others were saying about them. At the age of 35, I found out about kettlebells, because I had developed lower back problems from years of lifting heavy weights for athletics, so I began researching and learning all I could about them. Some people said they're bad for your back and shoulders. Some people said they're only a fad and their popularity would pass (except I found that they had been around for hundreds of years dating back to their first reference in Russia in 1704). Yet others swore by the benefits and feeling of youth and back problems disappearing by the daily use of the Kettlebell. People were raving about how they hadn't felt this good in years. People were actually getting more flexible and more powerful by the dedicated use of the cannonball with a handle.

This wasn't some invention on a late night infomercial that had been designed and engineered out of cheap plastic so that they could produce it for less and sell it for more. No. This was nothing but an iron ball with a handle. Simple concept: You pick it up, swing it between your legs, and voila`, you're on your way to a new you! Well, as I discovered over the years, the kettlebell's simplicity and our ability to learn its use fairly quickly does not mean an easy workout! However, it's been proven over and over that 20 minutes of safe and efficient use of a Kettlebell everyday will transform your body into something spectacular.

MY BACK PROBLEMS

Like I said earlier, I had back problems in 1995. I found out from regular visits to chiropractors that my Lumbar vertebrae #3, #4, and #5 were shifted slightly forward, causing pressure on nerves and the associated pain that goes along with it. Well, experts were not sure if it was degenerative, from a specific incident, or a little of both. Well, I can tell you with 100% accuracy that it's both. You see, back then I had a desk job, and I didn't have the best posture while seated and I was also performing very heavy squats for exercise, a very bad combination. On top of that, there was an ATV trailer incident (Isn't there always an incident?) I was moving my ATV trailer around manually by lifting up on the tongue and moving the trailer around in my driveway. However, on this particular day the trailer got away from me and started down the hill to the street. As you can imagine only bad things can happen with a runaway trailer. So I grabbed the trailer and stopped it from getting into the street and bam – *instant back pain*. After several visits to the chiropractor, with them telling me that I shouldn't be squatting with heavy weight anymore, and that my L3-4-5 are shifted forward, I wondered: "How am I going to stay strong without squatting 'heavy' and with a degenerative L-Spine?"

ANSWERS

Well, that's when I found the *girya* (Russian for Kettlebell) and became a *girevik* (Russian for Kettlebell Man). At this point in time, I was willing to try anything to alleviate the pain in my lower back, so I ordered the video "Enter the Kettlebell" by Pavel Tsatsouline, bought a Kettlebell and I embarked on a journey as a *girevik*. Amazingly, my back pain eased and eventually went away! For three years I trained with the Kettlebell performing all of the exercises I had learned without a bit of back pain! Because of that fact, I worked toward getting the courage and money to attend the Russian Kettlebell Challenge – a certification course put on by Pavel Tsatsouline in September of 2008. I was able to pass the certification course during that weekend and become an R.K.C. – A Russian Kettlebell Certified Instructor. The feeling of elation at the end of that course truly overwhelmed me and was very similar to when I received my first black belt at which time my Master told me this, "Your journey *to* the mountain has ended; now you must *climb*." I have since re-certified back in October of 2010 and will continue to 'climb the mountain.'

WHAT'S IN IT FOR ME?

Now, you're probably sitting or standing there wondering, "what can kettlebells do for me?" As promised, let's get back to the benefits of using a Kettlebell for fitness and why you should use them. Consistent & safe use of kettlebell exercises will:

- Literally melt the fat from your body
- Increase dynamic strength and muscle mass (Ladies don't worry – you won't look like the Governator, Arnold Schwarzenegger)
- Increase mobility and flexibility
- Increase mental toughness
- Improve cardiovascular conditioning

VIRTUAL FORCES

Because of a concept called "virtual Force," the nature of the "Hardstyle" Kettlebell lifts makes it so that you create forces much heavier than the stamp on the kettlebell. Because of this force, your body responds in a manner that develops a strength and resilience in you that no other piece of equipment can. Huge claims, I know, but having done it myself, I know it to be true. I have also seen all of my clients get stronger, gain muscle, lose body fat, and get into the kind of conditioning that they had back in high school. I have trained people ages 8-72 with Kettlebells with amazing results.

WHO USES KETTLEBELLS?

Secret Service members both in the U.S. and Russia use them. Special Ops Teams/Russian and U.S. Military use them. Professional Athletes, grandparents, schoolteachers, doctors, lawyers, middle & high schoolers, stay-at-home parents, executives, and anyone who is pressed for time can benefit from the Kettlebell.

In the Hardstyle system, we focus on functional movement not show muscle. Kettlebell training will develop your strength in all planes of movement and will get you into 'tip top' condition – lean and quick. Because of the shape of the Kettlebell, the weight is off-center causing you to focus on your balance. You will gain an increase in range of motion in your joints. You will have more resilience to injury because of this fact. We shouldn't work our bodies piece by piece. Instead you work your body as a whole, like nature intended. Hardstyle conditioning will develop your cardiovascular endurance exponentially because of the ballistic nature of some of the exercises. The benefits to our body's core will help anyone in everyday life, not just those who are high-level athletes. Fat loss will simply be a by-product of the Kettlebell work and you will reap that benefit immensely.

THE EXERCISES

The most common exercises are the 2-Hand Swing, Snatch, Turkish Get Up (TGU), Clean, Squat, and the Press. More advanced exercises are the Windmill, Bent Press, Push Press, Clean & Jerk, Pull-up, and Pistol. Each one of the exercises listed will utilize your entire body to some degree or another to perform them correctly. The foundational exercise, the 2-Hand Swing Proper is the basis for all other Hardstyle movements with a Kettlebell. This exercise will be the one that all individuals should begin with in order to develop the movement patterns for the others.

1. **2-Handed Swing:** The girevik begins with feet in an athletic stance maybe 2-3 feet apart with knees slightly bent. The Kettlebell should be on the floor out in front of the girevik in a manner similar to a long snapper in American football. This will be the starting point for all of the exercises. The girevik grabs the handle of the Kettlebell with both hands and essentially hikes the Kettlebell backwards and while holding onto the bell begins to drive their hips forward causing the bell to be driven toward the front of the lifter to chest height and then returning the bell back between the legs again in one uninterrupted motion without squatting or bending the knees too deeply. Breathing is of utmost importance and is similar to a boxer who is either taking a punch or throwing a punch. Thighs, glutes, and abs should be tight on the outward breath, which is triggered by the hip motion driving the bell forward. The inhale portion of the breath should be quick and deep as the lifter pulls the bell back between their legs. Doing swings for repetitions or for time will develop serious cardiovascular conditioning.

2. **The Snatch:** The girevik hikes the kettlebell back between their legs with only one hand and drives the hips forward causing the bell to be driven forward. Only instead of stopping at the chest, the bell continues up and above the head to an overhead lockout position. Shoulder down, lats fired, wrist straight, and arm even with or slightly behind the ear. Breathing is the same as the swing – as are the thighs, abs, and Glutes being tight. The snatch is the exercise that real hardstylers are tested with.

3. **The Turkish Get Up:** Lying on your back on the floor with the kettlebell beside you at shoulder level, you reach over with both hands and pick up the bell and push it straight up to a "firing range" position. Your same side leg is bent. You sit up to your opposite side elbow and then to your hand with the bell up over your head. You raise your hips as high as you can and pause for a moment so that you are on one hand and both feet. Then you bring your leg through to a sideways lunge position and then to a regular lunge position. Then you stand up. You come back down in the exact reverse sequence to the beginning position.

4. **The Clean:** Same starting position with the bell out in front of you on the floor. You hike the bell back between the legs and drive the bell forward with your hips, only you bring the bell up to your chest/shoulder. This is called the "rack."

5. **The Squat:** Same starting position with the bell out in front of you on the floor. You hike the bell back between the legs and drive the bell forward with your hips, only you bring the bell up to the rack

position. Now you simply squat for repetitions.

6. **The Press:** Get the bell to the rack in the same fashion as the Clean and the Squat. Only now you will press the bell overhead for repetitions to strengthen the shoulder girdle.

Remember in all the exercises above, the breathing is very important and so are the different stages of tension and relaxation in your glutes, abs, and thighs. Hardstyle strength and conditioning truly is a proven phenomenon and I will swear by it for the rest of my life and so should you. So the only questions left to answer are: When will you start your Kettlebell journey to the mountain? When will you begin your climb?

ABOUT VICTOR

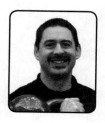

Victor Crawford was born in Alamogordo, New Mexico in 1970. He spent most of his life in Bloomfield, NM, where he graduated from High School. Victor received a scholarship to play Football at New Mexico Highlands University and graduated in 1993 with a B.A. in Business Administration/Information Systems with a Minor in Law.

He played college football, rugby, and baseball and has coached high school and youth sports for many years. He is a strength and conditioning consultant for multiple area high schools.

Victor has a Black Belt in Aiki-Jiu-jitsu, and has been training martial arts for 17 years. He is now an MMA coach with many fighters competing under his direction. He is into coaching, fitness training, and strength & conditioning. Other hobbies include camping, hunting and fishing.

Victor opened and operates a facility called The Body Factory, LLC in downtown Durango, Colorado which focuses on Kettlebells, Bootcamps, Kickboxing, Boxing, MMA, and Self-defense.

He is married to Michelle and they have two children, Myranda and Marcus. They are surrounded by forest and mountainous views at 7500 ft elevation in the mountains outside of Durango, Colorado.

Website: www.ViciousStrength.com
BodyfactoryDurango.com

E-mail: VictorRKC@ViciousStrength.com

CHAPTER 5

HOW I WENT FROM A "FAT BOY" TO A "LEAN, MEAN FIGHTING MACHINE"

BY ROB COLASANTI

I can remember sitting down at the dinner table at age nine and eating an entire pack of hot dogs by myself. I'd slice 'em up. Dip 'em in mustard. And chow down until they were gone.

Around this same time, I can also remember frequenting all-you-can-eat dives like *Duff's Famous Family Smorgasbord*. For $6.95, you could eat and eat and eat until you literally had to loosen your belt buckle on your way back to the car. Going in, the mission was always to "do some serious damage, get your monies worth and really tank-up!"

And that I did… After wolfing-down at least four or five heaping platefuls, piled high with an undistinguishable amalgamation of cheap, gut-busting buffet-style food, I'd aggressively segue into my favorite course of the entire marathon meal.

DESSERT!

Now, just for the record, I never approached the dessert counter like so many of the "sheepish" old ladies did. They were watching their weight (yeah, right) and therefore only snapped-up a few slices of peach, cherry or apple pie. Uh-uh, not me.

I'd attack the desert bar with "bad intentions," as we say in the fight game. For example, I refused to use those little, plastic ice cream cups that were sloppily stacked in crates next to the drippy, over-worked, soft-serve ice cream machine. I looked upon those things as "toys."

Me? I'd make my sundaes in the nice big salad bowls!

Oh, yeah… We're talkin' a tightly packed bottom layer of brownies…then a huge swirl of chocolate soft serve ice cream that extended all the way around the edges of the bowl…followed by a huge (but slightly smaller) swirl of vanilla ice cream…followed by a few hefty ladles full of chocolate syrup…followed by a few spoonfuls of each topping, ranging from nuts and sprinkles to cookie chunks and chocolate chips. And yes, I'd always put a cherry on top of the pile. (Okay, a few cherries.)

And for some odd reason, I always devoured my ice cream creations with a fork.

Anyhow, as you can imagine, I was a "Fat Boy," and as a result I was one of the most picked-on kids in school. I don't know – maybe eating like that was just my way of coping with the stress of a very difficult childhood. In retrospect, eating must have been my "escape."

EIGHT MONTHS OF MISERY

Then, at age 10, I was out riding my little brown bike one night, when I suddenly fell on the concrete. It wasn't a serious crash. But I was quite heavy and I landed just the right way…to break my left femur. (The femur is the largest bone in the human body. Not a good bone to break.) Next thing you know – I'm at the hospital, scared sick, in serious pain and being prepped for a body cast!

The hard, plastery contraption covered my entire left leg, half of my right leg and encased me all the way up to my solar plexus. There was a steel bar connecting my right and left legs at the knees. And, they drilled a steel pin all the way through my left tibia, which extended outward through both sides of the cast. I assume this was done to lock my lower leg in place.

Also, there was a hole cut in front for doing "number one" and a hole cut in the back for doing "number two." So for the next eight months, I laid on my back in front of the TV, watching mainly professional wrestling, wondering what the hell happened. Let's just say I got very good at using a bedpan, a 'piss' bottle and enduring lots of pain. Let me tell you, that body cast quickly became like a "prison" for me.

But it's a good thing my dad had a friend with an old, beat-up van. This enabled him to transport me back and forth to the hospital whenever necessary. They'd pick me up kinda like you'd take a pizza out of the oven, slide me into the back of the van, and off we'd go.

Eight months later, when I finally got out of the body cast, my skin underneath was a rancid black color and my muscles from head to toe had atrophied like those of an old man. Plus, I had to learn how to walk again. I went from a wheel chair, to a walker, to crutches to a cane, to a limp. My left leg ended up being one solid inch shorter than the right and remains so to this day. (Let me tell you, this is a real cross to bear.) But like most things, the whole broken femur episode eventually faded and I was finally able to walk again and get on with my life.

However, at age 11, I was now even fatter than I had been before I broke my leg. Why?

Because I had been laying on my back for approximately eight months, eating and getting absolutely no exercise at all. And when the body cast finally came off, I certainly wasn't ready to just spring into action. I was messed up physically and very overweight. I couldn't run, play sports or even do the basic exercises in PE class that other kids could do with hardly any effort at all.

I was constantly bullied, made fun of and treated like a total outcast at school because of my appearance, gait, cheap clothes and New York accent (my Dad and I moved to Florida when I was seven, so I still spoke like a New Yorker). Now there's only so much someone can take. Let's just say I was reaching the end of my rope. Yes, I was even contemplating suicide. And that's a pretty sad thing to admit some 28 years or so after the fact. But it's a reality.

MARTIAL ARTS...
MY WAY OF FIGHTING BACK

A few years had passed. By age 14, I was a good fifty or sixty pounds overweight, but fortunately I had become very interested in martial arts. I wanted to be a ninja! So I began practicing Ninjitsu in my backyard, by myself.

I used to take empty, one-gallon, plastic milk containers, fill them with dirt, tie a rope around the handle and hang them from the orange tree in our backyard. Then, I'd punch and kick the containers until they'd burst apart and all the dirt would come spewing out with dramatic effect. Felt good. Felt powerful...

Now, that's about the same time my across the street neighbor, Dan Masi, took notice of what was going on in my backyard. I guess our four foot high, chain link fence offered little camouflage for the so-called ninja in training. Dan mentioned to me that he was a black belt in Kenpo Karate. Upon recognizing my interest in learning martial arts, he volunteered to teach me some moves. And so he did, on and off, for nearly a half a year.

Then, one day Dan made a comment to me in passing. He said, "You should get yourself a heavy bag since those milk containers don't hold up very well." Me, being the type that I am, followed his "instructions" to the letter. So I persuaded my dad to take me up to Service Merchandise where I bought a 'big ole' red, Everlast heavy bag, using most of the gift money I had saved up. Oh, that bag was a big one – the biggest they had!

But now that I had the bag, I also had a challenge to overcome. There was nowhere, and I do mean nowhere, to hang that bag at our little house. So I came up with a great idea.

BLOODY KNUCKLES, SWEAT AND THE FIRST SIGNS OF WEIGHT LOSS

There was an elementary school located about a mile and a half away.

So I talked my dad into driving my bag and me to the school each night before dark. I would lug the bag across the field, and with Dad's help, I'd hang it from the monkey bars. Then my dad would patiently wait in the car, while I commenced to beating 'the hell out of that bag' ..."Rocky Balboa style," for as long as I could go.

No, I didn't wear boxing gloves. No, I didn't own a pair. No, I did not want any hand protection. I'd simply punch that bag as hard as possible, until my knuckles began bleeding. Then I'd keep punching and punching and punching some more. When the pain became too much to handle, or I completely ran out of gas, I'd call it quits for the night.

Then, my dad would help me unhook the bag and I'd lug it back across the field and put it back into the trunk. Next day, same thing.

Anyhow, this went on for many months and I had knocked off a good ten pounds beating that bag and sweating like a pig in the humid, Florida heat. Plus, I began doing various bodyweight exercises such as push-ups, sit-ups and pull-ups. This also helped accelerate my progress.

For the first time in my life, I began looking thinner and getting stronger. I was literally burning the fat off my body and my confidence quickly began to rise. Then one day Dan said to me, "I've done all I can do with you. You need to find yourself a karate school and a real instructor. You're ready."

"A school?" I responded. "Huh. Good idea."

THE NEIGHBORHOOD GOT A NEW LAWN BOY

I quickly found a karate school located not more than two

miles from my house. However, there was a problem right off the bat. The tuition was $470 for 18 months of unlimited training. This seemed like a fortune to me at the time, because I had no money.

So once again, I came up with a plan. Basically, I borrowed the money from my family.

But I had to pay the money back. That was the deal. So I borrowed my grandfather's little, red Craftsmen lawnmower and went knocking on doors. I literally became the neighborhood lawn boy and began cutting grass for $8 a job so I could pay back the debt. Or, for $10, I also weed-whacked the customer's yard. I didn't like doing this work, but it enabled me to fulfill my dream of learning real martial arts from a real martial arts teacher. I did what I had to do.

Now, I'll let you in on a little something...

I HARDLY EVER missed a karate class. In fact, I was at that school as much as, if not more than, pretty much anyone else. Why? First, it was because I truly loved the training. I took to it like a fish to water.

Second, I seriously wanted to GET MY MONIES WORTH! Frankly speaking, I had to bust my butt in the hot Florida sun and inhale massive amounts of dust, in the afternoons after school, and/or on the weekends, to pay for my lessons. I didn't get them for free like so many kids these days. So my training really meant something to me.

Soon I was cutting ten to twelve lawns a week. Plus, I was training at the karate school nearly every single day. Needless to say, the excess poundage I had been waddling around with for so long was literally melting off my body.

Then at age 15, I became a paid instructor in my martial arts school and eventually made my black belt in 1988. Then, I earned more degrees of black belt in the years to come, which was a very big accomplishment to make in a hardcore school twenty-something years ago.

End Result: I was a former "fat boy," who literally transformed into the proverbial "lean, mean fighting machine" for real.

TUNA, TUNA AND MORE TUNA

Around this same time, I adopted my own severely strict diet and dramatically reduced the portions of anything I ate. I cut out virtually all sweets, all sodas, all fried foods, all fast foods and all breads.

Pizza – OUT.
Birthday cake – OUT.
Pasta – OUT.
White rice – OUT.

I was incredibly disciplined for more than a solid decade. When I ate, it was almost always pure protein, fruits and vegetables. I drank mostly water and some coffee. Let's just say there were no more trips to the ice cream bar at Duff's. There was no ice cream, PERIOD! At that point in my life, food was NOT what was important to me. It was being a top fighter, an authentic black belt, a high-level martial arts teacher…and a guy who truly looked the part.

For many years, all I ate for lunch was two cans of tuna fish a day with some carrots, celery stalks or fruit. I'd open the tuna can with a handheld opener, drain the water off the top and then eat the meat right out of the cans with a plastic fork. That's it. No lie. No exaggeration.

One day while working out of my instructor's house, I stopped eating for a few seconds to answer the phone and his cat "Cali" decided to swoop-in and feast on my open can of tuna. "HEY! Get Outta Here!" I shouted. Then I quickly shooed her away and continued eating what was left, cause I was hungry and it was all I had with me to eat.

At the same time, I was training like an animal because my dream was to someday become a member of the United States Karate Team and win a gold medal in fighting. Or, to become the next Joe Lewis a.k.a. "The greatest fighter in the history of karate."

So, on Christmas day…I'd train first, then deal with gifts, family, dinner, etc. Before going out on a date…a three-mile run in the sun, with a sweat hood and sweat pants.

Super Bowl party…yeah, sounds like fun, but not until I work the bag for at least an hour, somewhere, anywhere… and with no AC.

My motto became, *"First we pay. Then we play."* I lived my life by this motto all day, every day, for many years. And that's simply how it was.

HELLO, 29-INCH WAIST!

Plus, I was teaching martial arts professionally seven days a week as a Chief Instructor, Program Director and/or Private Lesson Teacher. I was doing several thousand stomach exercises a week and at least a thousand push ups. (It may sound like a lot, but it's really not when you're teaching three or four hour-long karate classes every day, plus training yourself and others on the weekends, too.)

And Saturdays and Sundays were when I taught most of my

private lessons. I was consistently doing 10-15 per week for the extra money. My fee was a paltry $20 for one hour of instruction. And most of my private students came to me cause they wanted to fight hard, behind closed doors and with someone who could truly slam, or take them "to the edge." And frankly, I didn't care who they were, how big they were or what their background was.

I gave them what they paid for...and then some. After sending several students "too many" to the hospital (I went beyond the quota), my instructor banned me from sparring. He actually confiscated my fight gear, similar to the way a Police Chief takes away a cop's gun and badge. In retrospect, he did the right thing.

Bottom Line – I went from being a picked-on, little "chub-a-roo" to a guy who was breaking Louisville Slugger baseball bats in half with his shin in front of crowds of amazed onlookers. Being a bullied, laughed at, "fat boy" was truly a thing of my past.

And the only evidence I had left over from the fat-phase of my life was some nasty stretch marks, most of which I was able to conceal.

As a martial artist, my waistline remained at 29 inches for a good solid decade. And my weight had locked-in at around 140 pounds, though I was told by many of my instructors that I hit like a well-trained 200-pounder. In fact, my body had become remarkably toned and chiseled.

Once I went to see my doctor and she asked me to remove my shirt so she could listen to my heart rate. When I did, she looked me up and down, her eyes got big and round and she said, "Geez...what do you do for a living?" It just goes to show that Charles Atlas was right when he wrote about how a well-toned male physique quickly captures the attention of women.

Oh, my – what a turnaround I had made…along with the personal commitment to never be fat again, in this lifetime, or any other. But best of all, I had become a role model to others who also wanted to lose weight and get in shape.

Our martial arts school was extremely high profile due to the owner's expertise in the areas of marketing and publicity. Thousands of students came through our doors over the years and we even had a television show that reached a quarter of a million homes a week in the Tampa Bay area for more than a decade.

I was proud to have been a regular guest on the show. It gave me a small taste of what it was like to be a local TV star, since many of our students were regular viewers of the show before they joined the school. So I became a source of inspiration for many others (of all ages) who wanted to drop the excess pounds, become physically fit and eventually become a black belt, just like I did. In fact, all the instructors at our school were helping many, many students achieve their individual fitness goals through the unrivaled benefits of martial arts training. It was a beautiful thing! And then, my career took a very interesting twist…

WE HELPED COUNTLESS OTHERS LOSE WEIGHT AND GET IN SHAPE

In 1994, my martial arts instructor began an information business out of the spare bedroom of his house. He called it *The National Association of Professional Martial Artists (NAPMA)*. The thing truly took off like a rocket!

I became the first official employee and Vice President at the launch. Then, I had the honor of serving as the company's President from 2000 – 2008. To make a long story short, this company soon became the world's largest professional martial arts association. At its peak, the NAPMA organization had earned the business of approximately 2,100 active member schools representing more than twenty countries around the world.

Our popular World Conference became the largest martial arts business convention and trade show that the industry had ever seen up to that point. And, our magazine, *Martial Arts Professional*, was reaching 20,000 – 25,000 schools and instructors per month in North America. During its 14-year run, millions of copies – loaded with tons of quality information – were mailed to instructors throughout the country (and to our International membership base) for free.

This company generated tens of millions of dollars whilst I was a leader within it. But one of our most memorable accomplishments, which occurred in the late 90's, was when we launched Cardio Karate in tandem with Billy Blank's unbelievably successful Tae Bo program.

Cardio Karate was specifically designed to enable ordinary people to experience all of the weight loss and "get in shape" benefits of traditional martial arts training. However, it did so without requiring them to make the years-long commitment to earning a black belt, without having to wear a karate uniform and belt and without having to become a real fighter, or ever even get hit.

This program was light, fun, done to music…and it appealed mainly to women who wanted to burn fat, tone-up and get in the best shape of their lives. All total, we certified more than 6,000 martial arts school owners and instructors to teach Cardio Karate at their facilities throughout the country.

Plus, our organization inspired countless others to develop their own similar brand of martial arts fitness programming. So it is incalculable as to how many people experienced enhanced levels of fitness because of the movement we created and then supported for years. I just know the number is huge and I'm very proud that I was part of it.

IT'S TIME YOU CHANGE YOUR LIFE, TOO

Sometimes I pinch myself when I think about my remarkable journey. I went from being a "fat boy" with a broken femur, to an even fatter teen, to a "backyard ninja," to a lawn boy who cut over 1,000 lawns to pay for his karate training, to a tough-as-nails black belt with a 29-inch waist, and then on to become President of what was once the largest professional martial arts association in the country.

Not bad. Not bad, at all. So how did I transform myself from an overweight outcast to a highly respected guy who's interviewed all kinds of celebrities from Tony Robbins and Jackie Chan to Zig Ziglar and Jean Claude Van Damme? How did I become a guy who others now ask to have a picture with so they can hang it in their karate schools, or put it on their websites? How did I become an author? Speaker? Martial arts industry leader? Role model? How did I burn off so much flab, build so much muscle and confidence, and become so successful, when the odds were so greatly stacked against me?

Well, some of it had to do with being in the right place at the right time. I can't deny that.

But frankly, most of it had to do with hard work, uncompromising discipline, the ability to recognize and maximize good opportunities when they presented themselves, all combined with lots of serious unwavering determination to change my life for the better. Plus, I incorporated a no-nonsense diet and exercise regimen that simply worked wonders for me.

Once I reached my personal and professional goals, then my actions gradually became less and less about me, and more and more about helping others. This is one of the reasons I came to be known as *"The Ambassador of the Martial Arts."* Now, at age 41, I still wear 31-inch pants and I still do a little something every day to maintain my fitness. Most of the reason why I've been able to keep the weight off simply has to do with having a decent diet and doing some regular exercise.

My advice to you:

- Don't over-eat. Use portion control.
- Don't eat at night, after you've eaten dinner.
- Cut way back on sugar and unhealthy carbs. Aim for high protein.
- Drink lots and lots of good water and green tea.
- Stay away from processed foods as much as possible.
- And above all, exercise each day.

Also, remember this saying, *"Eat breakfast like a king. Eat lunch like a prince. And eat dinner like a beggar."*

Honestly, it's really not that hard to do all this once you make the commitment. And that commitment begins upstairs. <u>Success is 90% mental.</u> Once you change your thinking, you'll change your actions. When you change your actions, you'll begin to change your results. I did it…and I know that if you want it bad enough… then you will do it too!

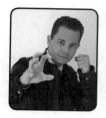

ABOUT ROB

Ambassador of the Martial Arts

Rob Colasanti officially began his martial arts training in early 1986 at *John Graden's USA Karate,* in St. Petersburg, FL. He borrowed his grandfather's red, Craftsman lawnmower and became the neighborhood lawn boy to pay for his first 18 months of tuition.

By the rank of green belt, he had already joined the school's professional staff. Then, for the next nine years, seven days a week, Colasanti worked in the trenches as a topnotch Program Director, private lesson teacher and Chief Instructor – as **USA Karate** evolved into a successful multi-school operation with an award-winning television show.

When Colasanti became the first official employee to the *National Association of Professional Martial Artists* (NAPMA) in the beginning of 1995, he was a young third-degree black belt with very little knowledge of how the industry worked. But through his dedication, integrity and passion, he quickly evolved into a respected industry leader, and eventually became President of the premier martial arts business association of the twentieth century – **NAPMA.**

He is the author of the book **The Martial Arts Business Bible**, which has been widely read by young instructors as well as many other industry leaders.

Rob Colasanti has broadened his leadership role as the one professional responsible for introducing the leading minds of business, sales, marketing and personal development to the martial arts industry.

His comprehensive interviews with brilliant and successful individuals such as Jackie Chan, Zig Ziglar, Anthony Robbins, Billy Blanks, Brian Tracy, Jay Abraham, Tom Hopkins, Matt Furey, Jean Claude Van Damme, Chet Holmes, Grandmaster Jhoon Rhee, Dr. Paul Hartunian, Benny "The Jet" Urquidez, Lee Milteer, Tim "4-Hour Workweek" Ferris, Joe Lewis, Bill Amelio of Dell Computers, Evander Holyfield, Bill "Superfoot" Wallace and many others have been hailed by thousands.

Today, Rob Colasanti has become recognized as the goodwill ambassador of the martial arts, and still maintains the martial arts skills and talents that launched his career.

He is no longer running **NAPMA** and *Martial Arts Professional Magazine*. However, he has emerged as a significant leader of the next generation of martial arts professionals, and is poised to become one of the primary forces to propel the industry to an even greater position of public prominence and respect.

Mr. Colasanti is helping to write the next chapter of the modern history of the martial arts industry, and the story of Mr. Colasanti's leadership and influence are destined to fill many more pages in the years to come. He may be reached at www.robcolasanti.com.

CHAPTER 6

FAT LOSS AND MUSCLE GAIN WITH ANIMAL MOVEMENTS

BY EDDIE BARAN

I f you've ever watched animals move, whether on TV or in person, you'll notice the power and grace they have. Whether it's their speed or strength, animals have the most incredible physiques.

But have you ever noticed something else about wild animals? They're all supremely lean and muscular. Not a single one is obese or even slightly overweight.

You might point to seals or whales, or even a grizzly bear and say, "They're not lean, they've got plenty of blubber." True, they do. But this is *functional fat*. They need this for survival, whether to keep warm or for hibernation, but it's not above what's natural. It's not fat due to poor diet and inactivity, like so much of the excess fat we see on human beings today.

I realize you might see a picture of a gorilla and argue he has a big gut, is fat and out of shape. Well, even though the gorilla's stomach might be large, he's not fat. The gorilla's big gut is mostly his intestines needed to digest all the plants he eats.

Perhaps you'll point to your pet dog or cat and tell me that he is quite plump. True, but domesticated animals are a different breed than animals in the wild. These animals are more "humanized" so their bodies reflect this.

The truth is that animals in the wild have a body fat percentage that is exactly where Nature wants them to be. They move in ways that keep them optimally lean and muscular. If they didn't, they'd die. There's no animal in his natural habitat that has too much fat, or fat that's detrimental to his own survival. ...except for the human animal.

THE DECLINE OF MODERN MAN

There was a time when humans weren't so fat. We were healthy, lean and vibrant. But with modern trappings like TV, fast food, processed foods, long days at work, hours spent in traffic, and worst of all – utter laziness and inactivity – modern human beings have turned into smaller versions of the Hindenburg blimp, with nearly the same fate. Yes, sorry to say it, but our society is 'crashing and burning' into deadly diseases like diabetes, heart disease, cancer and so on.

There has been a definite decline in our species. But what about the modern man or woman who does try to get lean and muscular? The person who does all the things he's told to do – yet still remains flabby and out of shape?

The truth is that most people are at a loss as to what to do. Look at any health club and the majority of clientele do not appear to be in shape.

The typical gym member usually quits due to boredom or lack of results; or he ends up spinning his wheels forever in hope of getting lean and muscular.

WANDERING IN THE DESERT OF DESPAIR

I ought to know because I was once the guy who trained and trained and never got the results he wanted. I wasted years lifting weights, hoping I'd get lean and muscular, but it didn't happen. I was either skinny and lean or muscular and flabby. But never what I really wanted: both lean and muscular. I felt like I was wandering in the desert searching for the answer.

I had always been involved with fitness from an early age, and was naturally skinny. Whether I was riding my bicycle for hours each day or lifting weights, I ate whatever I pleased and never had to worry about getting fat. Unfortunately I didn't gain much muscle either. I was your typical 'skinny dude' who couldn't gain fat or muscle. No matter what I did in the gym, I could never pack on any muscle size.

But this stopped shortly after I graduated from college. It was like my metabolism came to a screeching halt. And for the next decade, I gained a considerable amount of weight. I was no longer lean and I had a hard time getting used to this new squishy stuff on my body.

However, I did find it much easier to gain muscle. So I figured it was one or the other for me – either be skinny and lean or muscular with fat. By following a bodybuilding routine, I got up to 220 pounds. This was quite a jump from the lean 155 pounds I weighed when I started lifting. I'd like to say I was a shredded 220 pounds of pure muscle, but I had a lot of fat with supplement-bloated muscles.

By the time I reached my early thirties, I'd been consistently gaining flab that started to hang loosely off my body. Eventually I got so frustrated and confused that I just gave up on the goal of a lean and muscular build altogether, and focused primarily on strength training.

So I switched to power lifting because I stopped caring about how I looked and just focused on strength and size. My weight lowered to around 200, but again, although I had more muscle, I still had a good deal of fat on my frame.

After power lifting for a spell, I switched to Olympic weight-lifting. I enjoyed this type of training and I did lean out a bit due to the athletic nature of the movements, but I still had more 'blubber' than I wanted.

HOW A PAIN IN THE NECK BECAME A BLESSING

When the year 2000 came, I was fully immersed in Olympic weightlifting. At the time I had hurt my neck trying to strengthen it with some harness contraption, so I bought Matt Furey's *Combat Conditioning* program. I was only interested in his wrestler's bridge to fix my aching neck and had no interest in the rest of his program. After all, it was all bodyweight exercises – no weights, just you and your body. I dismissed this type of training because I thought calisthenics were for little old ladies, not a hardcore lifter and strong man like me. Boy, was I ever in for a shock.

The wrestler's bridge fixed my neck so well and made me

feel so much stronger, that I decided, just for kicks, to delve into the rest of Matt's program – to prove to myself I could easily do what he was doing. Imagine how shocked I was when I discovered I couldn't even balance myself in a handstand pushup position, much less do one.

I changed gears again, and dove head-first into body weight calisthenics. And as a result, my strength gains went through the roof, not to mention my conditioning and energy levels. Not only that, I also got something I'd wanted for years – a program that helped me lose excess flab.

Oddly enough, I didn't even care about whether I got lean from doing these exercises. I simply enjoyed the challenge they gave me, yet I was losing the flab I'd had for over a decade. I had pretty much given up on getting lean again, but now I was doing something that truly worked.

My neck pain turned out to be a blessing, because *Combat Conditioning* changed how I would exercise for the rest of my life.

From then on, I was sold on the benefits of bodyweight exercises and devoted myself to them. So much so, that in 2001, at the age of 35, I started studying gymnastics – the pinnacle of bodyweight exercises.

THE KINGS OF BODYWEIGHT

Gymnastics opened a whole new world for me because these athletes were the true masters of their bodies, the kings of bodyweight exercises. The gymnast was an animal athlete in the body of a human.

Although I loved this type of training, I wasn't a natural at it in any way, shape or form. I found it the most difficult training I'd ever done. It was frustrating beyond words, embarrassing, and at times humiliating. But I felt at home in the sport and was hooked.

After four years of training in gymnastics I became a gymnastics coach. Being a coach helped further my knowledge of strength, conditioning and movement. From my experience as a coach and athlete, I learned how the body worked on a much deeper level.

I felt more and more developed, like a wild animal swinging through the trees while doing gymnastics. I started identifying more with animals and how they moved in nature. When I kept hearing stories of how powerful animals were, I became even more fascinated. For example, I learned: How a chimpanzee could deadlift over 1,000 lbs. with one arm, how an orangutan could crush a crocodile with his bare hands, how a kangaroo could kill a predator with a single kick, or how an alligator could run on the ground at 20 mph!

From then on, I went on a quest to find out the hidden secrets of *animal athleticism* and how I could acquire it. It was the next logical step in my strength training. I researched the movement patterns of wild animals; I studied their behavior and anatomy; I trained the way they moved, adapting and improvising where necessary to get the results I wanted.

And the results were better than I could have imagined, and they happened fast. With this type of training, I dropped more fat from my frame, my abs solidified in unique ways, my muscles got bigger and more sinewy, my entire body developed into a more complete and efficient unit – I was functioning – and looking – more like an animal.

Best of all, I was getting leaner and more muscular without even trying. At the time, my only goal was gaining animal athleticism, yet more and more fat was flying off my frame and more muscle was replacing it. I was literally transforming my body into that of a beast.

I'd reached the point where I felt like I couldn't get fat even if I wanted to. The only way for me to get fat would be to quit doing these exercises.

This was what I had always wanted, but gave up on ever finding – a simple way to get lean and muscular. In order to find this ultimate fat-blasting and muscle building method, I had to wander the desert of weight training for 20 years to reach the Promised Land: the Jungle!

In fact, I was so sold on animal movements that I wrote three fitness programs on the topic: *Animal Kingdom Conditioning, Volumes I & II* and *Wild Animal Fitness for Kids.*

THE WAY OF THE ANIMAL

This *Way of the Animal*, as I call it, is exercising like an animal to get the benefits they get – lean and muscular, fit and athletic. So what makes animal exercises so effective in obliterating blubber and keeping it off for good? Why is it important for YOU to train like an animal?

These are the 8 top reasons why animal exercises are key in fat burning and muscle building:

1. Survival – Animals train for their survival. It's their instinct and natural behavior. Being lean is paramount for their survival because a fat animal is slow and won't be able to catch his food; or worse, he'll become someone else's. The human animal is no different. Too much fat is dangerous and will kill a human through deadly predators like diabetes, heart disease and a slew of other chronic conditions.

2. The most muscular movements – Animals are so much stronger, powerful, graceful, agile, balanced, coordinated, flexible, and conditioned than humans are – that it's not even close. So of course, that's whom we need to emulate. Their movements are the exercises we must model if we want to build muscle and burn fat. These compound movements use multiple limbs and joints. The more muscle you use, the more muscle you build, and the more fat you burn. There is no animal muscle developed in isolation. Can you imagine a gorilla lying on a bench press or doing bicep curls? No, he climbs, he walks on all fours. All of his muscles are being used in whatever he does.

3. Unique movements – Training like an animal is much different to how most humans train. Every possible angle and movement in the animal exercise repertoire has variety that is endless. This is not 'sitting on your butt' doing a 'pec deck' workout. This is putting your body in positions it has never experienced before.

4. Endless variety – With animal exercises, there is an endless variety of movements. This keeps your mind and your body from getting bored. When your mind gets bored, you won't want to exercise. When your body gets bored, you'll stop progressing; you'll adapt and your muscles won't respond anymore. It's impossible to adapt to all the varieties of animal exercises. This'll keep your mind and body guessing, continually *trying* to adapt yet never doing so. This keeps the workouts fresh and exciting and your muscles always fighting for stability, just like a wild animal in his natural environs.

5. Short workouts – It doesn't take much time to do animal exercises. Animal workouts are so intense and functional that your workouts will be shorter. You'll get much more 'bang for your buck.' No need to spend hours in a gym when a short 20-minute animal workout will do all you need.

6. Fast results – These animal exercises are so effective that they work very fast. Your results will come much, much quicker than with typical "human" training because the movements are unique and compound, so your body will use more muscle to do them.

7. HGH Generator – These compound movements not only build muscle and burn fat but they are great at naturally generating lots of Human Growth Hormone (HGH), your body's youth hormone that makes you healthier, younger, leaner and more muscular. This hormone is critical in getting you leaner and more muscular. Animal exercises load you up with lots of HGH.

8. Fun – Training like an animal is very fun to do. It's not even like you're working out; it's more like play. Like animals in the wild, in order to learn certain skills they play with other animals. In essence this is exactly what you will be doing with animal exercises. It adds great variety to your workouts. Some people don't like doing workouts with a certain structured plan of sets and repetitions. They'd rather go out there and move for distance or for time. Training for repetitions, time or distance is all valid and important, and training like an animal comprises all three ways. The more fun the exercise is, the more you're going to stick with it and see the benefits. One reason why gym training is ineffective is because it's so boring. Doing a leg extension machine, for example, is not only a poor excuse for an exercise, but it's dull and boring. No wonder most people quit going to gyms within three months of starting.

And the benefits to animal exercises don't end with losing fat and gaining muscle. You'll not only strengthen your muscles but also your tendons, lungs and heart; you'll sleep better, your energy will increase as will your flexibility. And these exercises will actually improve brain function. Research has shown that exercises that get you breathing hard improve your brain, and nothing can get you breathing harder than moving like an animal.

So let's start our journey into the jungle with the greatest animal exercise of them all… The Bear!

THE BEAR

The lion might be king of the beasts but the **Bear** is king of animal exercises. Of all the 36 animal exercises that are in my *Animal Kingdom Conditioning* programs, I consider the **Bear** the best of them all to burn fat and build lean muscle. It's simple to do and anyone at any level can benefit.

The **Bear** is the classic animal exercise. You'll see this done in martial arts and gymnastic classes, as well as high-level college athletic football and wrestling programs. It's one of the most effective exercises for developing all-around strength and conditioning. This exercise is perfect for all fitness levels and is usually the place to start if you're a beginner. And if you're advanced, this will take your body to pure animal supremacy – fit, lean and muscular.

This exercise is a great way to indoctrinate you into the world of animal workouts. This should be among the first animal exercises that you do. Go slowly at first to get used to the position, as it will be new to you. In gymnastics it's one of the first exercises we teach young children as a way to get them used to being on their hands and strengthening the upper body. But it's also an excellent conditioning exercise for the legs, lungs and abs.

1. Get on all fours, hands and feet on the ground.
2. Put your rear end high in the air. Arms and legs should be slightly bent. You can place your legs wide or narrow. Try different widths.
3. Now walk on all fours by alternating your hands and feet.
4. Breathe deeply.
5. Go as far as you can without stopping or getting up.
6. If all you can do is one step at a time then that is fine. Begin there and build up.

After you get good at moving on all fours, the next step is to pick up the pace. Instead of walking, start jogging or running in the **Bear** position. This will improve your balance and your muscular and cardiovascular conditioning. Make sure you can do the **Bear** correctly before trying to move faster.

BEAR PROGRESSIONS

According to your level, you'll be doing the **Bear** in different ways. Start with the Beginner progression and move up from there. Here are the steps to make sure you're advancing correctly. You don't want to overdo it and go too hard at first.

Beginner – Get in the **Bear** position and walk as far as you can before you need to stop, even if it's for only a few yards. If that's too difficult, hold the position for as long as you can to get used to it before advancing to walking. When you can **Go Bear** for 50 yards without stopping, move on to the intermediate level.

Intermediate – At this level you will move a little faster and farther. Work on going for a longer time without stopping. When you can get to 75 yards walking fast you're ready for the next level.

Advanced – Now you're going to go even faster and farther. You should be running fast. When you can do 100 yards without stopping you have really accomplished something! You can even sprint 100 yards if you're really feeling brutal.

BARAN'S BRUTAL BEARS

Here's a great example of an animal workout that's fun to do and very effective in building muscle and burning fat. And it takes very little time. I call it **Baran's Brutal Bears**, because that's what they are: ferocious killers of fat and slovenliness.

It consists of just the **Bear** exercise. Where it specifies rest, make sure you fully recover between each set. You want to have enough energy to move. Take as long as you need to get your heart rate steady. You should be breathing very heavily at the end of each set, not at the beginning. The short bursts of interval training are key for building muscle and losing fat.

1. 15 seconds – Bear sprint. Rest and recover.
2. 15 seconds – Bear sprint. Rest and recover.
3. 30 seconds – Bear sprint. Rest and recover.
4. 30 seconds – Bear sprint. Rest and recover.
5. 45 seconds – Bear sprint. Rest and recover.
6. 45 seconds – Bear sprint. Rest and recover.
7. 60 seconds – Bear sprint. Rest and recover.
8. 60 seconds – Bear sprint. Rest and recover.
9. 45 seconds – Bear sprint. Rest and recover.
10. 45 seconds – Bear sprint. Rest and recover.
11. 30 seconds – Bear sprint. Rest and recover.
12. 30 seconds – Bear sprint. Rest and recover.
13. 15 seconds – Bear sprint. Rest and recover.
14. 15 seconds – Bear sprint. Rest and recover.

You can do this workout three days a week. It will take about 15-20 minutes to complete. If you find this too tough, then substitute half of the Bear sprinting with Bear walking. If this is still too difficult, then cut the workout in half and work your way up to the full version. Remember to go at your own comfortable pace.

Now that you've been introduced to animal movements, you will be entering an exciting new world of exercise – a wild world that's fun, fast and effective. You will start feeling the effects of this animal training immediately. You will see visible results in a short time, as your body will become more animal-like, leaner and more muscular.

Welcome to the jungle! Now go out there and have fun burning fat and building muscle the Animal Way!

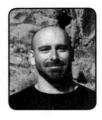

ABOUT EDDIE

Eddie Baran's specialty is showing men and women of all ages and abilities the unique, effective and fun ways to become much better athletes. He has been involved in fitness for almost thirty years. Growing up in San Diego, California, he was your classic skinny weakling, but always had an interest in strength and exercise.

He dabbled in lifting weights for a brief period then stopped. In his late teens, Baran rediscovered fitness as an endurance athlete, becoming a road cyclist typically logging in three to four hour rides each day. He later resumed weight training, doing bodybuilding routines. Baran hopped onto the bodybuilding and weight training bandwagon hoping to get massive.

For the next decade, Baran continued on his bodybuilding quest, bulking up from a lean 155 pounds to a puffy, pumped-up, supplement-bloated 215 pounds. Although big, Baran was hardly strong and definitely not a conditioned athlete. Realizing he was all fluff and no substance, and that bodybuilding was not about functional strength, Baran began training in Power Lifting, which eventually led him to the Olympic-style weightlifting in which he went on to compete. But he hungered for more conditioned-based strength routines.

Baran was the first ones to begin training with Matt Furey's **Combat Conditioning**. He made such tremendous gains in strength and conditioning, and was so excited about how effective bodyweight exercises worked, that in 2001, at the age of 35, he decided to start training in gymnastics. Along with Furey, Baran coauthored **The Secret Power of Handstand Training** and **The Primate Power Super Strength System**.

Baran continues to this day to study gymnastics. His gymnastics coach was so impressed with his understanding of gymnastic fitness that he asked Eddie to help him coach the sport, specializing in strength and conditioning for recreational and competitive gymnasts – ranging in ages from 8 to 18.

His fitness programs include **Body Sculpting Bodyweight Exercises for Women**, **Wild Animal Fitness for Kids**, and with his brother, Andy,

Gymnastic Abs, **Gymnastic Handstands** and **Animal Kingdom Conditioning I** & **II**.

Eddie Baran can be reached at: **www.EddieBaran.com**.

CHAPTER 7

SUPERHUMAN FITNESS MADE SIMPLE

BY VALERY FEDORENKO

What if I told you that by reading this short chapter, you would have the knowledge to bring yourself or someone you love to Superhuman Physical Status? Maybe you have never heard of this term "Superhuman" or think of it as something mystical or not real. First, let me explain what I mean when I say Superhuman, and then I'll show you how you can be one too. Did you catch that? I said how you can be one "too". Yes, that means I'm referring to myself as a Superhuman, but before you dismiss what could be a life-changing moment for you and call me arrogant, this is what multiple people have said about me since I was a teenager. When you hear something over and over again from different people for 20 years, you will tend to start believing it too. The thing is, I know it's nothing genetic, nothing unique to me, nothing really special at all except an understanding. I'm not a freak, a mutation, an error or an evolution. I get sick like you do, ...I feel pain just like you do, ... and I have fears just like you do. I think my average, or even below-average youth made me seek out a way to cheat the system and not only get even, but get ahead of others. I stumbled upon a secret Superhuman Training Method because I was bullied, made fun of, and worse, as a child. In fact, as a Junior Athlete I broke an all-time Men's record. That means not only did I do something no other Junior had ever done, but I did something no other HUMAN had ever done. This is what I call Superhuman. Also, I want to point out that I stumbled upon this understanding, but I could not stumble if I didn't take the first step. I had a reason. I went looking for an answer. I believe now that I have that answer and can share it with you. In fact, it is my work. Sharing this understanding with others is what I do now with my life.

Superhuman, to me, does not mean something alien, or "of the gods" like the ancient Romans or Egyptians might have thought. It's not a Superhero fantasy read out of a comic book or seen in a movie. Remember the Bruce Willis movie Unbreakable? He was the sole survivor of a huge train wreck where he didn't even sustain a scratch. Come to think of it, he had never been seriously injured, EVER, despite playing football and having been in a major car accident earlier in life. He had not even been sick. Oh, there was one time he almost drowned, but that of course was his Superhero weakness. They all have one, as you know. That's not me. I have been injured in accidents and I have been beaten up. I've sustained broken bones and been through surgeries as a result of these things. I have the scars on my face to prove it. I'm not Mr. Glass, but I'm not unbreakable either.

WHO AM I?

I guess it would only be right to formally introduce myself since you are about to hear my secret but simple method to Superhuman Fitness. I'm Valery Fedorenko, a Strength & Conditioning Specialist born in the former USSR in 1973. While I am proud of many things I accomplished, such as becoming World Champion, breaking World Records, and attaining the sport ranking of Honored Master of Sport, the most rewarding thing for me was immigrating to the USA in 1999 and introducing the Russian Kettlebell to America. So by now you can guess that my tool of choice for Superhuman Fitness is the Kettlebell. Maybe you've even heard of the Kettlebell by now, since it's in almost every gym, on TV Infomercials, and even sold at Wal-Mart, but I'd like to give you my impression of this tool.

WHAT IS A KETTLEBELL?

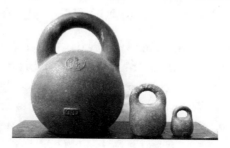

The original purpose of the kettlebell was an official weight for a scale, not a tool for Fitness.

The classic kettlebell is basically a precision weight with a handle on top for ease of movement. I have an 1870 version that is a little more than 32 Kilograms or 70 lbs. and the size of a bowling ball, but there are some of a similar date that are just grams, and as small as a golf ball. Who invented the first kettlebell is unknown, and is probably similar to asking who invented the wheel. We do have examples from ancient Greece of brass kettlebells of various shapes, and there are drawings that likely represent kettlebells in Egypt and China that probably make the origins prehistoric. In the Olympus Museum, there are specimens of shaped rocks that were used in the

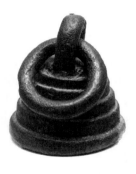

games, so even though they were not used for sport or fitness the same way we use them now, the mere sight of a handle on a weight begs someone to lift or throw it. Russians just

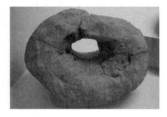

perfected the Kettlebell, what I call the Modern Kettlebell, and adapted it for use in Fitness. The difference in comfort between a classic kettlebell and a modern kettlebell is like night and day.

WHAT IS A RUSSIAN KETTLEBELL?

The Russian Kettlebell has standards. Leave it to the Soviets to make things official, but that's probably the best thing that every happened to Fitness and, for sure, the best thing for Kettlebells. With standard measurements in the height of the kettlebell, the circumference of the ball and the diameter of the handle, you can now have a sport with World Records and numbers to compare yourself to. Americans and Europeans had something like a kettlebell over 100 years ago, maybe more, but these aren't the same as a Russian Kettlebell. Maybe you've seen them in old Strongman photos? Basically these are ball weights with a handle screwed in. Not good for what I use the kettlebell for. I have heard these called Handleweights or Handlebells, but those fell out of favor 100 years ago for a reason. You can't do much with them! Many of the kettlebells you'll find sold and in use today have been corrupted by the Fitness Industry "experts". Funny shapes. Bad handles. Poor quality. Buyer beware! The simple fact is they just don't have the insight to create a kettlebell based on performance.

They do it anyway for two reasons:

1. They want to have a "unique looking" kettlebell so they can establish their brand. As you know, if a star puts their name on a product, it really doesn't have to be a good product in order to sell well.
2. They completely bypass the main feature of the Modern Kettlebell, which is uniform dimensions, no matter what weight – for the sake of price.

Note that Modern Kettlebells used for Fitness are the same size, no matter if you use weights of 8 Kilogram or 48 kilogram. The lighter ones are hollow. The shape is determined by the human body and how the kettlebell fits you. The trajectory you will lift them in remains the same, so why would you want to change size as you progress with your lifting? You would not. It's cheaper to make a kettlebell that is solid, but small, bigger, BIGGER, and HUGE! You know, they look like the Russian Nesting Dolls, we call Matryoshka. These are toys in my opinion. They call this product classic kettlebells, but you aren't weighing produce at the market, you are doing Fit- 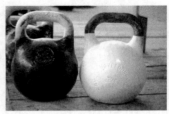 ness. You are about to become Superhuman with this tool! Don't settle for less. Get a Modern Kettlebell.

WHAT BENEFITS CAN YOU GET?

Sit down. Get ready for this. Maybe you won't even believe

it because it sounds too good to be true, but Kettlebells can enhance every part of your Fitness. Officially, traditional Kettlebell Sport that I once competed in professionally more than 20 years ago is categorized as Special-Endurance, but there are other ranges of time and other uses of Kettlebells that prove to enhance Power-Endurance, Strength-Endurance, Strength, Power and Endurance all at once. I'm going to say without reservation that this tool is the most powerful single tool you could have to enhance yourself physically. You might be able to find something equal to it, but not better. You can certainly use it along with other forms of Fitness or other tools, but if you had to have just one thing to whip you into shape and keep you there, the Kettlebell cannot be beaten. I take it even further and say this tool develops all the official components of Physical Fitness – such as Metabolic, Bone/Joint/Tendon/Ligament Integrity, Morphological, Muscle Strength, Muscle Endurance, Body Composition, Cardiovascular, Flexibility, Agility, Balance, Reaction Time, Power, Quickness, Speed, Coordination, Mental Toughness, Emotional Health, Mental Sharpness and also generalities such as Well-being and Health.

WHAT'S THE SECRET?

The secret to Kettlebells is quite simple. First we start with basic human movements that involve the whole body as a unit. I will tell you now that it is possible to get extreme Fitness with just one or two key Kettlebell exercises. If someone told me I had only one exercise I could do for the rest of my life, no exceptions, I would choose the Kettlebell Snatch, but there are many you can choose from that will give dramatic results, and give them fast. Exercises such as Swing, Clean, PushPress, Jerk and LongCycle are great in their own right, and if you take a few of these, or just one, and make progress in time/distance, reps-per-minute (RPM) and weight, and tie these simple concepts in with technique and logical practice, you will have no choice but to change who you are physically and even mentally, all for the better.

> *"A complex system that works is invariably found to have evolved from a simple system that worked... A complex system designed from scratch never works and cannot be patched up to make it work. You have to start over with a working simple system."*
>
> ~ John Gall in *Systemantics: How Systems Work and Especially How They Fail*

In all my athletic endeavors, even the ones recently that were not Kettlebell related, I have always approached them with the mentality that the fastest and most simple method to reach my goal, one that doesn't get me hurt, is THE BEST! I'm fairly opinionated about that, but it's really an individual thing to a certain extent. For one thing, your goal or your extreme may be completely different to mine, and it probably is. We all have different things we bring to the table, such as past injury, current health or lack of reliable information. My goal is not to tell you what your goals are. My goal is not even to tell you exactly how you have to get there. My goal is as simple as the methods I employ and the concept with which I did what I did in the past and what I do now, which is to bring you the truths that I have discovered through my own extreme practice with this simple tool. This is the tool THAT YOU CAN USE to find your own best way for yourself.

The movements themselves are not extreme. It's your choice how far you want them to take you! Your body is designed to PUSH and PULL. The ballistic nature of the exercises, coupled with multiple repetitions that get the heart pumping and the lungs expanding, make Kettlebells an all-in-one, one-stop-shop for Fitness. Of course, I must advise you to seek the counsel of your health care provider before you begin any exercise program, and I'd also advise you to learn as much as you can from someone you can trust for ANY new activity, but what I do know about Kettlebells is that many, many, people can at least accomplish the movement required to get some benefit from this tool. Nothing is absolute, and if you have some major disability that prevents you from doing kettlebell movements, then I'm truly sorry for having wasted your time. Hopefully you still can learn something that would benefit someone you love by reading this.

However, I believe in the wide accessibility of Kettlebells. For example, I had a student come to one of my Kettlebell Coach Certification Courses that was over 400 pounds! They actually had problems just walking. Keep in mind, this is the course where people come to prove to me that they are capable of duplicating my information and worthy to be called a World Kettlebell Club Coach. Some of these people are Professional Coaches and Trainers, working with UFC Fighters, as well as players from the NBA, MLB and NFL, and of course, University and High School Athletes and in Gyms around the world. We have Coaches from all branches of the Military, Police and Rescue. In fact we have certified over 1100 people in just a few years time, some of whom are just Kettlebell Enthusiasts, that now have the knowledge of my techniques and methods for themselves, their friends and family or clients. I'll admit I was skeptical that this tool, even with the knowledge I had of it, was the right choice for someone that had problems with "normal" movement. I thought maybe they would be better off in a pool or maybe with something else. Still, I gave them a chance. Guess what? I was wrong! Even though they had trouble walking, they could do Kettlebells! I was surprised and inspired all at once. One of the new revelations with Kettlebells that my Russian brothers didn't realize is the fact that we stand in one spot and perform exercise that can be taken to extremes, that can also be used by people with ambulatory problems! I'm happy to say that this student above passed the course and is now a WKC® Coach.

BECOME SUPERHUMAN IN 7 SIMPLE STEPS!

It is my opinion that Kettlebells can bring a human to their potential physically. Of course there is no question that you are going to have to actually use this tool. Sitting it in the corner is not going to get it done! You never will hear me talk about easy. You may hear me talk about fast or powerful or Superhuman when talking about Kettlebells, but you are going to have to sweat and breath hard and endure a little discomfort to find this superhuman that lives deep inside you. Also, I didn't really talk directly about weight-loss, as I believe this tool and these methods go far beyond just the appearance aspect of Fitness, but you are going to have a hard time holding on to fat if you do this long enough. In fact, Kettlebell Lifters have an amazing metabolism. I never really worried about the types of foods I ate, although I have always eaten a simple and natural diet.

Sometimes, especially when I was competitive in the Sport of Kettlebell Lifting, I would wake up in the middle of the night with my body just asking for food! I finally got smart and just put food next to my bed. I didn't even have to open my eyes. I'd just wake up, reach, and eat. I'm not suggesting you start doing that the day you begin Kettlebells, but listen to your body. After some time you will become who you really are. Fat will come off, bones will get stronger, you will become more flexible and strong, and even your skin will improve. You will be tired in the beginning from all the new stimuli you are putting yourself through, but you will soon be so full of energy that you will not even understand what's going on. I'm not a doctor, but I feel my organs are working better when I am stable in my kettlebell workouts. I even feel my mind is sharper. So, I wish the same feeling for you but it's something I really can't put completely into words. I hope that you will try and give it some time to work for you. Below are my 7 simple steps that I feel are most important in how you approach becoming superhuman by way of the Kettlebell.

STEP 1:
ACQUIRE THE RIGHT EQUIPMENT.

It should go without saying that I do not recommend a kettlebell from your local discount department store or sporting goods shop. It seems the bigger the chain the worse the kettlebell choice. Still, if you really want to get started, I guess I would prefer anything that resembles what I consider a kettlebell over nothing at all. I'm just telling you up front though, that you are wasting your money, and you could be setting yourself up for injury. I have designed my own Kettlebell called the VF Prograde™ Kettlebell, the highest quality kettlebell money can buy. This is the standard by which everything is measured now across the world. It's a Russian Kettlebell, or "Modern Kettlebell", in that it meets all the competition requirements, but it has been designed further to be the most comfortable kettlebell ever made. I've made this model available for years, and it is likely the most sought after and copied kettlebell design ever made. I'm proud that people finally understood the classic kettlebell with a big fat handle and various sizes of ball is better left for the farmers market and not for use as a Fitness tool. I'm also proud that many have tried to counterfeit my design too. It's the best form of flattery! Wait until everyone sees my newest designs though! As I'm writing this I have just released my new Performance Kettlebell™ System and also five new designs! This system will feature a sophisticated bevel or relief area for the arm to rest comfortably against. You see, comfort is important in Kettlebell Lifting because you must endure, and you don't want something as simple as pressure on the back of your arm to stop you. This addresses this completely! This is revolutionizing Kettlebell Lifting, whether it is for Fitness or Sport, across the board. It's probably the single most important improvement since the "one size for all weights" standard that the Soviets implemented 60 or 80 years ago. My newest designs will all keep the logic of one size for all weights, but each type of Kettlebell, or the intended use will be a different size. For example, we have a new Standard Competition Model, with contours. We also have introduced a Womans Competition Standard, which also has the contours.

While it's smart to have one size so as you progress in weight everything else remains the same, it always bothered me that women had to live with this standard. What I didn't tell you before is the Soviets, when designing the standard, took average measurements of men, not humans. They didn't really count the women into the equation because women weren't into Kettlebell Sport or really much Fitness then. Times have changed, even in Russia. What I did was simple. I took average measurements of women and made a standard that is more appropriate for them. There is also a contoured model for Fitness, that is even a fraction smaller than the Womens Competition model, but it has vinyl protection over the metal to make it more "gym friendly". I have also made an adjustable kettlebell model that allows for greater portability in the field, adjusting from 12kg to 32kg, and the SuperHeavy Kettlebells that go up from 52kg into the stratosphere of kettlebell weights. Basically if someone can lift it, we will make it! Generally, I suggest a woman start with an 8kg, and a man might want to start with 12kg. I'm proud of my new designs, especially the introduction of the Performance Kettlebell™, and you can only get them at: http://store.worldkettlebellclub.com

STEP 2:
PRACTICE PERFECT TECHNIQUE.

I can't emphasize enough the importance of technique, in anything that you might do, not just Kettlebells. Don't fall for the excuses that people, even supposedly high-level Trainers, come up with. They say, "that's just technique", as if it's somehow not anything else. Like magic or what? A trick? No. I know Strongmen that bend wrenches and horseshoes, and while they do practice technique, they are REAL strong. I assure you that a professional Boxer works on technique constantly, but they can really hit hard, no trick, no gimmicks. I'm sorry to tell these Trainers that people who have been past where they have been know the secret. Technique is supremely important to real strength, power, endurance, speed and in my opinion, everything Fitness. When someone tells you to make something harder, and that it really is so that your body adapts to this more difficult way, you should run and not look back. Every real athlete attempts to make things easier, period. We have many ways to make things harder. Trust me, you can make it as hard as you want or need by always working towards making your Fitness easier. If you want to accelerate your technique in Kettlebell Lifting, I suggest becoming a Member of World Kettlebell Club® and acquiring my Instructional Video: *Intro to Kettlebells – THE Essential Quick Study™.*

STEP 3:
INCREASE WORK CAPACITY.

Now that you've learned technique to the point you can execute the exercises safely, you must work to get your capacity up. This is an important transition. Most people when starting Kettlebells find out very quickly that they have a work capacity problem. Work Capacity is a simple concept. It's your ability to work and keep working. Some people are really strong, but can't keep going for more than a few minutes. Some are not all that strong, but their endurance is good, however they still have problems sustaining work because they are not strong enough or resilient, and they break down and have to stop. There is no other way around it. In order to approach Superhuman status with Kettlebells, you are going to have to bring up your overall Work Capacity. There may be a point that you can't even sweat with the use of kettlebells because you stop before you even sweat. Trust me, if you keep working on your capacity by adding sets to your workout and increasing the time you do these sets, you will get to the point where you could even get an extreme workout with just one set! I'm at a level now that I can maintain a very good capacity with just one long, hard set, three or four times per week. It's the fastest workout anyone could ever wish for, but in order to get to this point you have to pay your dues and get your capacity up, which will take a little time.

STEP 4:
PUSH THE REPS.

After you've learned technique so you can safely begin to increase your sets and total work capacity, you could begin to 'up' the repetitions. Increasing reps is the main factor for superhuman performance. Life is about reps. Why does the military drill in long hikes in boot-camp? Why do Fire/Rescue Services make recruits pass stair climb tests? Why does the Police Academy put a lot of focus on running for their new officers? Virtually every sport team puts a sharp focus, if not a total focus, on high rep activities. There is a reason. Yes, over the last several decades, especially in the USA, a push for low rep or even max rep lifting, even for Fitness, has become popular, but Coaches and Trainers are returning back to reps due to injuries and out of necessity. While their athletes or personnel are getting stronger, it doesn't do much good if they are injured, immobile and lack much needed endurance. Kettlebell Lifting by way of reps has made me resilient, athletic, fast and powerful. What's interesting is nearly 100 years ago the old-time Strongman George F. Jowett in his book *The Unrevealed Secrets Of Man* had it right. He spoke of extremely strong men, record breaking, circus show types, who got that way by lifting light weights, usually not more than 25 pounds, and he was talking about lifting for strength and power in the back and legs, not the biceps! The point is, he believed in training the "Mental Impulse" and never to the point of failure. We do this by adding reps, one by one. We do this by over and over sending the right message to your nervous system and muscles, tendons and MIND! We teach ourselves to contract and relax, contract and relax, to a great degree and with precision. This is real strength and something that cannot be beat!

STEP 5:
GET YOUR WEIGHT UP.

No, I don't mean your body-weight! That's almost certainly going to go down while you get stronger, more powerful and gain endurance. What I'm talking about is increasing the weight of the Kettlebell. I don't suggest you get greedy and try to lift heavy Kettlebells. After you learn technique and continue to practice technique, after you increase your work capacity, after you increase your reps, you will feel when it's the right time to increase the weight of the Kettlebell. Every time you make a true improvement in Conditioning that allows you to increase the weight of the Kettlebell, you will inch closer and closer to Superhuman status. I started lifting with a 16kg Kettlebell when I was 12 years old, and now looking back, it was too heavy for me. I didn't have someone guiding me at that point, but luckily I didn't hurt myself and just kept going. I tried to lift more every day! By the time I was in my late teens, I was lifting that same weight and much more for hundreds of reps without sitting the kettlebells down. Recently, I broke my own record with a 60kg Kettlebell (132 pounds) by lifting it 70 times without putting it down. Steady progression works!

STEP 6:
DON'T EVER QUIT. UNLESS...

This is a mentality thing. If you truly want to get to Superhuman status, you never really stop pushing yourself. You can change your focus, work on other Kettlebell lifts, or even other forms of exercise that are at least congruent with your overall quest to become Superhuman, but you should not stop. So many times people reach to a fairly high point in their training, but are either too afraid of such a high status of Health and Fitness that they "change strategy," or they simply get complacent and their progress halts. They are on the edge of Superhuman status and don't even fully understand it! Now, I cannot tell you how far you want to go. I can only explain to you the steps I took to achieve Superhuman status, and offer my opinions on how you can do it too. My advice is: use this information to get the level of Fitness and Health you desire, and then maintain it. If my words and experience help you in any way accomplish that, then I have achieved my goal for you. That being said, you must listen to your body. I have had very few training-related injuries in my life because I really take care to not work past my current condition or capacity. If your technique starts to break down, stop! The goal is to have the first rep look the same as the last. If you feel any injury, don't push through. See a health-care professional and get it checked out. You should also go back and re-evaluate the above steps, as something must have been rushed. Either your technique needs improving, or you got greedy and increased the weight too quickly, or you did not let your body repair itself with enough nutrition and proper rest. Remember, we are all human working towards Superhuman status. There is no magic. It's real adaption over a period of time! Enjoy your experience as you learn about yourself, and above all, you are doing this to be healthier and happier.

STEP 7:
GO TO EXTREMES!

OK, so my last bit of advice is the last step, and something you may not fully understand until you make your way through some of these first steps on your journey to Superhuman status. In fact, you can't fully understand what I'm talking about when I say go to extremes, until you master all the previous steps. Now that my tendons, joints and bones are Superhuman, I can take myself to extremes. Now that my muscles and lungs are ready for just about anything, I seek something I haven't done and prove to myself I can. I now pick a new goal, maybe thinking months ahead or even a year or more, and I accomplish it. I try to think of something extreme, as general Fitness or even competing in Sport are not things I'm concerned with at this stage. I want to be healthy and happy too, but I feel that when I'm working towards something exciting automatically. I never work towards a goal that makes me unhappy. I do this and always learn something that I can then pass on to Members of our Club. I have never recommended anything that I have not tried, almost to extremes, myself.

So, I wish you an exciting journey on your way towards your own Superhuman status, whatever that may be for you. Please visit my YouTube Channel for additional free tips and insights: http://Youtube.com/VFWORKOUT and see some of my personal interests these days. But don't let it scare you off! Some of these clips are extreme feats and not at all how I recommend you start. Come visit us at the World Kettlebell Club, sign up for our newsletter and get started the right way now!

ABOUT VALERY

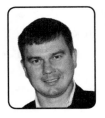

Valery Fedorenko is a World Champion kettlebell athlete from the former USSR who has records still standing after more than 20 years. A subject of early Soviet Sports Science study, Valery was the first Kettlebell Expert to reveal his methods of super-fitness to the public. Even though he does not compete today, he stays in top condition using his own form of Strength and Conditioning by way of the Kettlebell, and has dedicated his life to bringing that information to other athletes as well as those looking for a simple form of fitness that promotes health and well-being – and at the same time produces results.

Along with the organization World Kettlebell Club®, Coach Fedorenko multiplies his information exponentially by producing WKC® Master Trainers that are authorized to transfer the specialized knowledge and methods to other Trainers. Those Trainers go on teaching their own students and so on. The lineage within WKC® is unparalleled in the industry. It's not uncommon to see a WKC® Champion who is Coached by a WKC® Champion who is also Coached by a WKC® Champion. World Kettlebell Club® literally has the top current athletes from around the world as part of its team. Valery Fedorenko has been called the Worlds Ambassador to Kettlebells.

Coach Fedorenko has personally worked with UFC Fighters, NFL Players, MLB Players, and many other Pro and College Athletes, as well as Police, Fire and Military. He continues to Coach a few Kettlebell Athletes, but he prefers to instill his methods of super-fitness in regular people who had no idea what potential they had within them.

To learn more about Valery Fedorenko, find him on YouTube and Facebook @ VFWorkout.

CONTACT INFO:

Facebook.com/VFWORKOUT
email: VFWorkout@gmail.com
ValeryFedorenko.com
WorldKettlebellClub.com
service@WorldKettlebellClub.com

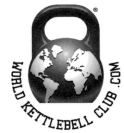

CHAPTER 8

WALK AWAY…TO BETTER HEALTH AND FITNESS

BY CHRIS VILLAFANO

As a preteen and teenager, I was always about 30-50 lbs overweight. I realized at about 15 or 16 years old that I no longer wanted to be overweight. At the time I started out by working out in the gym like every other teenage guy and lost some of the weight. But as an adult still battling weight issues, and one who lost his father to diabetes complications, I knew I had to get into shape. For me the gym wasn't always feasible, so I needed a plan I could follow to get into shape one step at a time without gym membership fees or the time spent there.

What has come from my personal quest for weight loss and fitness is a walking routine for the average person – real people, not the ones you see on television spending hours at the gym with their personal trainer. I have developed a walking fitness plan that you can do anywhere and achieve results. What I am sharing with you here are the key things I have found that really work – to walk your way to better health and fitness.

1. WEAR THE RIGHT SHOES

I have personally been wearing some of the new shape and tone variety of shoes. They are great for this type of exercise. Several companies make these new shoes made to tone your legs while you walk, but the important thing is to get the right fit and comfort for you. Any shoe designed for walking will do the job. If you do decide to get the new shaping variety, please remember to practice walking in them a bit on terrain you know. You will need to get used to the feel, and rough or unfamiliar terrain is not the best place to break any shoe in.

2. SELECT A DIET PLAN

To maximize your weight loss as you walk your way to fitness you will want to select a diet program that works for you. Eating the right foods in the correct quantities will get you healthier faster, and allow your body to be the calorie burning machine it was meant to be while you walk.

3. USE YOUR ARMS

You aren't supposed to resemble a tin soldier with your arms at your sides while you walk! Get your arms moving too, not just your legs. You can use hand weights while you walk to do punches, military presses, bicep curls or tricep dips as you walk. You can even do shoulder shrugs to tone your back and shoulders while you walk. Why should your legs have all the fun? Don't feel like carrying weights with you?

You can start as I did, in the rainy season, with an umbrella in your hands. Carrying something with you, even something as simple and lightweight as an umbrella, can help get your arms into the action. Walking offers the advantage of being able to do more arm exercises than running will allow you to do.

4. KEEP A JOURNAL

A journal will allow you to track both your eating and your exercises in one place. There are some great fitness tracking programs online or for your phone, but you don't have to get that complicated! Get a notebook and start journaling. You will want to track what you ate, how many minutes and where you walked, as well as what exercises you did for you arms on your walk. Track how many reps of each exercise you did. Track your warm up and cool down exercises too. This will help you to not only see where you have been in your new health plan, but it will allow you to see what is working.

5. WEIGH YOURSELF DAILY

I know that some of the health and fitness specialists, and even the diet plans, recommend weighing yourself only once a week. Personally, I need the accountability of a daily weigh in. You might want the daily reminder too. Remember that this is designed to keep you on track, not as a reason to beat yourself up over it. Weigh yourself in the morning, before you eat or drink anything so that you will have a consistent record of where you stand with your weight. You can track this in your journal as well.

6. DRINK WATER, DRINK WATER, & DRINK WATER

Start your morning with a glass of water with lemon to flush your body. During the rest of your day, you will want to consume a minimum of 6-8 glasses of water. Add 2-4 more glasses depending on how much you sweat during your walks each day. You should be drinking water before every meal as part of your 6-8 glasses per day. Studies show that drinking water before a meal will actually promote weight loss by making your body eat less and feel full faster.

Should you bring water with you on your walk? I personally do not carry water with me on my walks because I am only going for 30 minutes or so, and I have had my glass of water with lemon prior to my walk. There's nothing worse than being on your walk and needing to find a restroom either. However, if you are in a warm climate and feel you need the water with you, take small sips as you are walking. Drinking too much water along the way can give you cramps and slow your pace.

7. WARM UP AND COOL DOWN

Before you begin your walk, you MUST stretch. Here are some simple stretches that I encourage you to do before you walk: calf stretch, quadricep stretch, hip stretch, Achilles stretch, hamstring stretch, kneeling quad stretch, squating adductor stretch. Any stretches that you do not know how to do can be found on the internet. The temptation is there to jump out of bed and just head out for your walk. If you are using hand weights during your walk you must remember to stretch your upper body as well. Do some head circles to stretch your neck muscles.

Begin with a 5 minute slow-start, warm up walk. Progress to the brisk "bring on the sweat" walk. After your walk you need to slow down and cool down for about 5 minutes. You should stretch again upon completing your walk.

How Long to Walk? How long should you walk? Long enough for you to re-charge your batteries!

Isn't it funny that we take the time to charge our cellphones or our laptop computers but we often don't allow time to re-charge our own bodies? You need to walk for 20-30 minutes at least at a brisk pace. This doesn't include your warm up and cool down time.

Are you afraid you can't take the time to walk? Consider this multi-tasking solution. When I go for a walk, I put a load of clothing in the washer. By the time I get home, the clothes are ready for the dryer, so I just did two things at once. Afraid you might miss your favorite TV show – you can DVR the TV show, but you cannot DVR your life! If you are a morning news watcher, watch the news while you stretch and get ready for your walk. You can always fit walking into your life.

8. WHEN TO WALK

Learn to be a morning person! Walking in the morning offers some advantages over walking in the evening. When you walk in the morning you get your exercise out of the way instead of dreading the thought of it all day long. A morning walk offers you time to focus yourself and to plan for your day. Plus, since you want to work up a sweat while you walk, your morning walk will mean you won't have to squeeze in an extra shower during the day. Wake up, stretch, walk and then shower is the perfect way to start your day. In a way, walking before you start your day is even environmentally friendly because you will save water by only having to shower once.

Wait. What if the kids or an early work-start time will keep you from walking in the mornings? Don't worry, you can walk any time. You can walk on your lunch hour or in the early evening when you get home from work. But please note that it is not a good idea to walk within the hour prior to going to sleep. Brisk walking can really amp up your system and make it difficult for you to achieve proper sleep. If you go to sleep at 9:00 p.m. then ideally your walk should be completed with cool down no later than 8:00 p.m.

9. HOW FREQUENTLY TO WALK

I suggest you walk 20-30 minutes everyday if possible. If that is not feasible for you, then you should get at least five days of walking every week. If you are busy and you cannot plan when to walk, realize that you can walk anywhere! You can park further away at work or at the store and walk a greater distance to the door. Don't beat yourself up if you miss a day or two. Start walking again the next day. Slow and steady will win this race.

10. TRACK HOW FAR YOU WALK

How should you track how far you walked? Get a pedometer. A pedometer will allow you to track every step you take – everywhere. You can count your steps walking up the stairs at work or at home, count your steps at the mall or at the beach; you can count your steps pushing your child in the stroller. You can even count your steps on the treadmill while watching your favorite movie. Make it your goal to try to achieve 10,000 steps a day!

11. DRESS FOR THE WEATHER

If you walk in a climate that can change quickly, as I do, then you will want to be prepared for the weather. It is important to keep your body warm and well protected from the elements as you exercise. Wool vest or shirt or thermalwear in colder climates are good. Rain gear to stay dry is important in wet weather too. In cold weather don't forget to keep your head covered and to wear gloves. There are some great products out there now that transfer moisture to keep you dry and comfortable during your walk. But avoid cotton blends when it is wet because once they get damp, they will stay damp. And remember appropriate socks to keep your feet dry and toasty. To really rev up your workout you might try a sauna suit which is ideal in the 60-70 degree temperature range, but be careful that you don't cause yourself to overheat!

What about those people who live in really warm climates? You need to dress for the weather as well. You don't want to overheat or promote chafing. Comfortable, well-fitting walking clothing will help keep you comfortable. People in any climate should remember to use sunscreen. When you return from your walk and shower, consider using aloe-based lotions as part of your routine to replenish moisture lost as you sweat the weight off in the elements.

12. AVOID MINOR INJURIES

Dressing appropriately and warming up beforehand should help you reduce minor discomfort and injuries, but here are a couple things that can help just in case. Blisters can be caused from ill-fitting shoes or the wrong socks. If you get blisters, soak them in Epsom salts and cover them with a bandage. Rashes can happen, especially on inner thighs. Two things work really well to avoid rashes: Spandex compression shorts like bicyclers wear and anti-chafing balms such as BodyGlide will help keep chafing to a minimum.

Even walking sticks or Trek poles can assist you in staying injury free. If you are walking along uneven terrain, a walking stick will help give you more sure footing while also giving you something to carry to help give your arms a little workout.

Use lip balm. Whether in the warmer or cooler climates, you need a lip balm with sunscreen for two reasons. You need to protect your lips from sun exposure and the wind, and also you will be breathing through your mouth, which tends to dry out your lips.

13. HEALTHY FOODS AND SNACKS

I am a big fan of low calorie snacks that also help your body. Celery is a great source of fiber, fills you up, and burns more calories as you chew than it actually has in it. Lower carbohydrate foods will help your body lose weight as will whole grain foods. You should be eating lots of vegetables and salads at least once or twice a day. Drink skim milk for calcium and no fat. Pineapple is a high fiber source that will satisfy your sweet tooth. Banana is a great source of potassium which your body needs during exercise and loses with perspiration.

14. SAFETY TIPS

Wear bright, reflective colors especially if you will be walking at dawn or dusk when visibility is low. Walk on well-lit roads and paths. Avoid uneven ground or areas with potholes or broken pavenment – an ankle turn can force down time where you will have to start all over. Be aware of your surroundings. Stay out of the way of traffic. Pick a path that is away from vehicles whenever possible. Don't let your ipod become a safety issue – you cannot drown out all of your surroundings and still stay safe.

Where you walk is not as important as to just start walking. If you live near the beach and find it restful or more exciting to walk on the beach, then do it. If you have to be at the football field for your child's sports practice and you want to walk on the track there, great! If you can't stand the idea of walking in the weather or where people can see you, then walk on the treadmill at home. No matter where you choose to walk, you will have made a great decision for your health.

Walking may be a low impact exercise, but you can make it a high impact workout and get high impact results. Walking is self-paced. Don't worry if you can't walk a mile the first day. Can you make it around the block? No? Well then try to walk to the end of your street the first day. You can always add a few steps or the distance to the next driveway tomorrow.

Remember the words of the Chinese philosopher:

"A journey of a thousand miles begins with a single step."

~ Lao-tzu, (604 – 531 BC)

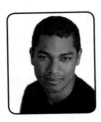

ABOUT CHRIS

Chris Villafano is a graduate of Lamar University in Beaumont, TX. He obtained his Bachelor of Science in Communications with an emphasis in Film and a Theatre minor. Chris was a proud member of Student Support Services, Lamar Filmmakers Association, and the Fine Arts Film Society.

While attending Lamar University, he acquired numerous awards in the Communications department and Student Support Services. He became the first Student Employee of the Year (2009).

Chris is no stranger to publication. Besides being on the Pulse 2008 editorial staff, Chris's poems, "The Battle of Glutton" and "Tender Soles" were selected in that publication. He also worked in the Student Government Association, campus library, radio and TV station.

Outside of Lamar University, Chris has been involved both in front of and behind the camera, working variously as actor and Executive Producer from time to time.

Chris has been an active member of Toastmasters, winning several awards and certificates of completions. In addition to his other accomplishments, Chris served as Sergeant at Arms and Vice President of Public Relations.

CHAPTER 9

3 SECRETS TO SOUND SLEEP

BY STEVE GRZYMKOWSKI

T ruth be told, I never had a problem falling asleep or staying asleep. Didn't matter how much sleep I got either; I'd wake up feeling completely rested.

In fact, I could lay my head down on the pillow and be out in seconds. At home or traveling…hot or cold temperature, light or dark in the room… it didn't matter; Mr. Sandman came to me in seconds. That guy sleeping on the airplane through all that turbulence…that was me. Boy, it used to tick my wife Chris off!

Then one ordinary Friday night, my youngest daughter, Sophie, crawls into bed with us. This was something Chris and I became accustomed to over the years with raising 4 kids. The usual routine was for me to put the kids back into their beds as I always could fall back asleep after such disturbance and my wife couldn't. Sounded like a great plan, never mind that my wife had to wake me most of the time to put the kids back to bed. I somehow missed the logic in her plan but nevertheless went along with it.

Oh well, where was I? Sophie crawls into our bed, I wake and look at the clock to see it's 1:00 am. For some reason, this night I just rolled back over and went back to sleep...not returning my daughter to her room.

Next, I'm abruptly awakened by my daughter shaking at my back, I look at the clock, it was 4:45 am... she must be dreaming, I thought. I called her name for her to stop, but it continued. At this point, my wife and I were both awake and I turned on a light. Sophie was having a seizure.

Being in the medical/pharmaceutical field, I've seen my share of health-related events. This was the most frightening thing my wife and I have ever experienced. She came out of it after what seemed like an eternity, when in reality it was about 45 seconds, we rushed her to the hospital and they ran the gamut of tests. All tests came back normal, and we were sent home after being told that 95% of kids will have one seizure and never have another. Sophie had 2 more seizures that day.

As you can imagine, the nights that followed were pretty sleepless. Sophie slept in our bed the first week and we were up at every twitch and whimper. When we moved her back to her room we went ahead and installed a video monitor. This was supposed to give us peace of mind so we could rest, but the sleepless nights continued. Needless to say, one sleepless night ran into the next and before you knew it my wife and I were weeks into it getting by on little or no sleep.

We were physically and mentally exhausted. I tried keeping

up with my exercise routine but it was spotty at best. Now this, coupled with a normal exercise routine is a recipe for disaster. Our bodies, your body, needs rest in order to rejuvenate itself...add in an exercise regimen with no sleep, and you are not doing your body any good – especially if you are not getting a full 8 hours of sleep. It's a fact backed up by boatloads of literature and studies: A good night's sleep is key to your losing weight and burning fat. I knew something had to change.

I took this time to monitor myself to see what I was doing now, compared to what I was doing when I could fall asleep. Many of you may say that it's obvious why we weren't sleeping and who could blame you under those circumstances. And you'd be right, but millions suffer from insomnia and broken sleep, and those people's circumstances can't all be like ours, something in their lives has caused them to suffer from insomnia or broken sleep.

I didn't stop there; I also researched what the body does during sleep and why the body needs rest. I was shocked to find a recently notorious hormone, HGH, was involved.

Human Growth Hormone? Could that be the missing link in your exercise routine? Well, yes and no. It plays a part in the missing link. And yes, I'm talking about the same HGH pro athletes are paying someone to inject them with, except I'm not advocating you go out and get HGH injections. Instead, I want you to produce it on your own. No, not in your basement. Get it the old fashioned way...from your very own body.

Yes it's true...your body produces it and you're probably wondering why you need HGH...especially when it gets such bad press. In my opinion, the bad press is because of the consequences of injecting yourself with something that's not natural.

Many of HGH's benefits are well documented; it reduces fat accumulation, it builds lean muscle mass, it has anti-aging properties, and many athletes were taking it as it improves endurance and increases energy. And I didn't even mention that it helps your immune system. Don't believe me? Go ahead and Google "HGH's benefits"... I'll wait.

Do you know how you can get good old-fashioned HGH from your body the natural way? I'm talking maximizing the levels your body produces so that it'll burn fat right off your body and build lean muscle mass. The answer is REST... more specifically Sleep.

Sleep... Good quality, uninterrupted sleep and what happens during sleep; that's the *Missing Link* in your exercise routine.

Getting a good night's sleep allows your body to repair and recharge itself – physically, mentally, and emotionally. It is nature's way of healing your body. And your body produces the most HGH when you are in a deep sleep.

Throughout the remainder of this chapter I will give you three exercises, rather, *3 Secrets to Sound Sleep*, that'll assist you in bringing your mind and body to rest before you go to bed. These are the same exercises I developed to get myself and my wife back to sleep after all those months of sleepless nights. Exercises that will help you achieve the deep, uninterrupted sleep your body craves. The kind of sleep that'll put your body in a state to produce the most HGH it can... naturally.

SECRET #1

I cannot stress this enough, you were born with the ability to sleep... your parents laid you down and you went to sleep. Not until you knew the stresses of everyday life did you find difficulty in getting to sleep. Sleep, or lack of sleep, is most often caused from one thing... your mind and body not being at rest.

And here's what I discovered: when I was awakened by a noise on the monitor, my mind would begin to race... almost transporting me back to the very day my daughter had her seizure. This thought led to another disturbing thought, and before you knew it, I had memories popping back into my head that had nothing to do with the initial event. The mind would race.

Imagine if you will, a very large steep hill, covered with the whitest of snow. On top of the hill you stand with a snowball in your hand and roll it down the hill. As it moves down, it gets bigger and bigger... growing larger, almost taking on a life of its own... snow piling on it that wasn't part of the original snowball... just getting bigger and bigger.

This is how my mind raced during this period of sleeplessness I went through. I imagine its how your mind gets during those nights you find yourself lying in bed, wide-awake.

So I realized a very important secret, if I could focus my attention on one thing... and not let any other thoughts into this focus, I fell right back to sleep with ease. So I developed what I call the "Chalkboard principle."

You must wipe your mind clean before climbing in under the covers... write down the various "I can't forget to do this tomorrow" thoughts... get them all out of your mind then lie down. Your mind will naturally begin to relax itself, knowing that you've written down important tasks and knowing you've prepped for the next day. Now begin to think of one thing, or recite one thing in your head over and over again... soon you will be asleep.

SECRET #2

Now, if you have no problem falling asleep yet find you wake up in the morning tired, not completely rested and wanting to go back to sleep, then you must ask yourself one question. Are you pre-programming your mind for a bad night's sleep?

What do I mean by this? Well do you inadvertently put certain parameters on yourself before retiring for the night? I say inadvertently because you might not even say these things out loud but you may be thinking them.

Things like "I must get 8 hours of solid sleep or I wake up feeling horrible," or "if the room's too hot (or cold) I won't be able to sleep; how about "if the doors open then the light will come in and wake me," and even... "I have never slept well when I travel or in hotel rooms."

Henry Ford once said, "Whether you think you can, or that you can't, you are usually right." The same applies to getting a good night's sleep. This is called auto-suggestion and its something I used to do all the time not realizing what I was doing. When you talk like that to yourself, your body is just obeying the programming you are giving it.

So all you need to do is to *RE-PROGRAM* your body.

Instead, set different expectations of your night of sleep. Let's try it; "I'm going to get to sleep and wake up happy and refreshed, revitalized and ready to tackle the day." Come up with whatever suits your situation, just make sure it's the right programming.

SECRET #3

Gifts of the Magi

When we hear the words above, we typically think of the three wise men that followed a star to the baby Jesus. The three wise men were also called Magi, and what many don't know is that this ancient tribe of wise men brought much more than the three gifts of Gold, Frankincense, and Myrrh.

Those were the three gifts they brought on that night...on other nights they passed down ancient secrets to their loved ones...exercise secrets that were passed from generation to generation. Secrets that would help cure certain illnesses and disorders.

Many of these secrets were never written down, and like most things they became lost over time, thought to be gone forever.

But in my search of literature surrounding insomnia and getting sound sleep, I rediscovered these lost secrets of the Magi. I'm going to share three of the sleep inducing exercises with you. By no means are these strenuous exercises, but I recommend that you first consult with your physician before adding any exercises to your regimen.

1. The First Position: Strengthening your lungs

Standing, your heels should be in line and close together, the knees held back and the toes turned out at an angle of about 60 degrees. Then, with the body straight and inclined forward, so that your weight falls on the arch of the instep, you are supported by the toes and only lightly on the heels.

Your arms should hang tensely from the shoulders. Your hips should be a little drawn back, your chest advanced, your shoulders square, the head erect and your chin slightly drawn in while your eyes are looking straight to the front. In each hand, tightly clasp a hard rubber ball as this aids in keeping the muscles rigid. If you prefer you can simply close the hands tight, so that the muscles become tense.

Lift your arms until they are parallel with the floor; hold the hands so they are facing downward. Make all the muscles of the body as rigid as possible. Take a long breath in through the nose and hold it for a few seconds, then exhale by contracting the abdomen as much as possible. Repeat this twice, first with the hands facing downward, then follow with them upward, then downward, and upward again.

Relax your muscles and drop your arms parallel with your body. If at any time you feel tired, stop for a few seconds; then continue the exercises with your mind centered.

2. Drive out the stress

Take the first position. Clasping a rubber ball tightly in each hand; extend your arms horizontally at right angles with your palms facing up. Keep your muscles rigid and your upper torso thrown slightly forward. Now as you inhale, lift your arms slowly upward until your hands meet over your head. Tighten the muscles in your entire body for a few seconds while holding the breath.

As you exhale through the mouth, lower your arms slowly to your side, keeping your muscles rigid, forcing the stress out of you. This is an excellent exercise to reduce stress.

Inflate your lungs as you bring the hands upward and exhale as you bring them downward. Repeat this exercise eight times. I like to think of clean pure air as I inhale on this exercise, relax, and then drive out the stress upon exhaling.

3. Last one to prep you for a great night's sleep

Lie flat on your back, either on the floor or in your bed. Put your hands under your head.

Keep all the muscles of the body rigid and take a deep breath, not too rapidly, expanding your lungs to their fullest extent. Hold the tension for a few seconds, and then exhale until your lungs feel perfectly empty. Release the tension as you exhale.

Repeat this 10 to 12 times unless it makes you dizzy. If so, do not take such a deep breath until you can get accustomed to this exercise.

I look forward to hearing from you regarding your success with the *3 Secrets to Sound Sleep.*

For the complete *3 Secrets to Sound Sleep* Program, which has DVD's detailing the exercises above along with other exercise "gifts from the Magi," please visit us at: www.thesecrettosoundsleep.com

To see the life-changing relationship and parenting products we have, please visit us at: www.thefamilyaffect.com

ABOUT STEVE

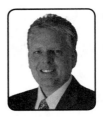

Steve Grzymkowski was born in the small town of Manchester, Connecticut. In 1983, at the age of 16, his father's job promotion relocated the family to Pennsylvania. Distraught over being uprooted, he confided in a girl he met at the school bus stop. She too moved into the neighborhood a year prior under similar circumstances. Over the final 2 years of high school, they shared stories, found comfort in each other, and became good friends. A few months after graduating high school they began dating.

Steve Grzymkowski now lives in beautiful Bucks County, Pennsylvania with the girl from the bus stop ... his lovely wife Christine, who not only happens to be his high school love, but also his very best friend. Together, they have four wonderful children, Emma, Evan, Olivia and Sophie.

Steve is first and foremost a family man, as you can see, but he is also a self-made man with a solid sales and marketing background. He has escalated through the ranks to the top of his field, winning numerous awards within his industry. Steve gets noticed, not only because of his likeable personality and wonderful sense of humor, but also for his smarts in the real, common-sense business world. Exclusive Think Tank organizations have taken notice of Steve's talents and have asked for his involvement on various high-level projects. You may actually know of Steve through his various publications on Marriage and Parenting, being somewhat of an authority on family and marital matters.

Steve's interest in Physiological exercises has brought him to where he is today. Only scratching the surface of potent sleep methods in his now out of print book "3 Secrets to Sound Sleep", Steve set out to discover the lost secrets of the Magi. And he unearthed a treasure trove; a system of exercises with the power to relax and induce sleep.

To learn more about Steve Grzymkowski and the "NEW 3 Secrets to Sound Sleep Program" please visit: www.thesecrettosoundsleep.com

To learn more about Steve's publications on Marriage and Parenting please visit: www.thefamilyaffect.com

CHAPTER 10

HOW TO EAT DESSERT AND STILL LOSE WEIGHT AND GAIN MUSCLE!

– ENJOY COOKIES, CHOCOLATE MILK, AND OTHER SWEETS

BY JEFF STREU

We've all been there before: it's the holidays and there are a bunch of cookies and other goodies lying around. Do you just eat a small amount each day and hope it doesn't go to your waistline? Do you gobble them all down so that they're out of your sight? Or do you deny yourself and avoid them until you crack and end up binging? I've done all three of these things before, and although the friend or relative that gave them to you was just being kind and generous, the cookies certainly aren't too nice to you.

So how do you make all of the desserts disappear? You could just give some to others, but you'd probably like to enjoy some yourself, right? Fortunately there is a way to eat sweets and not gain fat, feel guilty, or feel deprived. In fact, when done properly, they can help your muscles recover from workouts.

As a senior in high school, I was cutting a lot (possibly too much, but that's a different story) of weight to wrestle at the 103 pound weight class. I was managing my weight well, through disciplined training and eating, but I was dreading the seemingly inevitable weight gain that accompanies the holidays. Being that Thanksgiving, my birthday, Christmas, and New Years all fall during wrestling season, I was bombarded with junk food and treats for practically a month. In previous seasons I buckled under the strain of a strict diet by overindulging during these holidays, and the pig outs came with a price. Being that I was cutting more weight than ever my senior year, I realized I needed to keep things under control.

During my junior year I came across a helpful hint, and that was to eat a small amount of sugar immediately after working out to help your muscles recover. What's more, none of the sugar would get deposited as fat, either; if ingested right after a workout, the sugar will go directly to the muscles to refuel them. It seemed too good to be true since I was of the mindset that junk food should never be in a wrestler's diet, so I started off by having some fruit right after practice. I figured that I should stick with a better form of sugar. In high school practice ended at 5:30, but I usually wasn't home for dinner until after 6:00. For the first few years I didn't eat or drink anything during that half hour, except possibly a little water. As a result I would be starving, exhausted, and dehydrated by the time I ate dinner. This small change improved my recovery and energy after practice tremendously.

As I geared up for my final high school season, I decided to be a bit more advanced with my recovery methods. I had since found out that sugar plus a small amount of protein works even better after a workout than just sugar, and so I tried some Accelerade™ and Endurox® R4®, two sports drinks known for their 4:1 ratio of simple carbohydrates to protein.[1] They tasted great after a workout and made my muscles feel even greater.

When the holidays rolled around I put this technique to the ultimate test by treating myself to some guilt free dessert after working out. I recall eating jell-o, cookies, cake, pie, and more during the Christmas break. Since I let myself indulge a little, I didn't feel any cravings, and the best part was that *I didn't gain an ounce.*

The Accelerade™ and the Endurox® R4® worked well, but I eventually realized how much money I was spending on them. Luckily I had found out a cheap and delicious alternative: chocolate milk. It has roughly the same ratio of carbs to protein as the other drinks, making it great for recovery after workouts. There was a fellow student who sat at the same lunch table as me my senior year who was lactose intolerant, and so he always ended up throwing away the milk carton from his school lunch. Rather than see it go to waste, I gladly took it from him and saved it for post-workout. Once I got to college I took full advantage of the unlimited meal plan at the dining halls by making sure that I got some chocolate milk after wrestling or going to the gym. It never made me gain weight; in fact, maintaining my weight seemed even easier than ever, and I felt like I had boundless energy.

---

1 <u>The Science of 4:1</u>. PacificHealth Laboratories, Inc. 5 January 2011
  <u>http://www.accelsport.com/product-info/Accelerade-4-to-1.html</u>.

So who wouldn't like to have a big glass of chocolate milk every day while losing weight and building muscle? Before you get started, there are a few guidelines to remember to make it work correctly.

1. **Immediately following a workout** – In order for the sugar to feed your muscles instead of going to your waistline, you can't wait until you've driven home from the gym, showered, changed, etc. The magic time is twenty minutes after the last repetition is finished. Thirty minutes is pushing it, but is acceptable. When sugar is consumed within this time frame it will go directly towards refueling your muscles and helping them recover. When taken after the twenty to thirty minute mark, your muscles aren't nearly as starved for glycogen and so some of the sugar will be stored as fat. Anytime inside of those twenty minutes will do, but the sooner the better. Ideally, you'd want to bring your recovery drink to the gym in a water bottle or a shaker cup if you are mixing up some powder. Of course, if you are using chocolate milk, put it in an insulated bottle or a small cooler so that it doesn't go bad during your workout.

2. **Intense exercise** – You can't get away with eating sugar after just any workout. In order for the sugar to feed your muscles, the muscles must, to a certain extent, be depleted of glycogen. After a session of high intensity running, biking, swimming, or strength training, or hard training sessions of wrestling or other sports, your glycogen levels will be at a low, and so the sugar

will be used as immediate fuel.[2] Activities such as yoga, walking, stretching, etc., although good for you, won't get you huffing and puffing or burn glycogen the way that high intensity exercise will.

3. **Consume protein with sugar** – Traditional sports drinks contain only simple carbohydrates and electrolytes. However, it has been shown that sports drinks with a 3:1 or 4:1 ratio of carbs to protein are even better for recovery after workouts. Chocolate milk is perfect because it falls right into this range. I also sometimes make my own recovery drinks by mixing Gatorade® with whey protein in the proper proportions, which is very similar to what most store-bought recovery drinks are. If you have a blender you can try creating your own combination of carbs and protein by throwing in some fruit, yogurt, milk, protein powder, honey, peanut butter, you name it. Note: when purchasing recovery drinks or making your own, be aware of any artificial ingredients that might be tossed in as well. Although effective, many recovery drinks or powders have several fillers that probably shouldn't be in your body.

4. **Liquid is best** – Although a banana with peanut butter will do the trick, I usually prefer to have my recovery meal in liquid form. Not only will liquid foods be absorbed into the bloodstream faster, but they will help rehydrate you as well. I like to weigh myself before and after wrestling practices to know

---

2 Karp, Jason R., Jeanne D. Johnston, Sandra Tecklenburg, Timothy D. Mickleborough, Alyce D. Fly, and Joel M. Stager. "Chocolate Milk as a Post-Exercise Recovery Aid." International Journal of Sport Nutrition and Exercise Metabolism. Volume 16, Issue 1. (February 2006). Human Kinetics Journals. 5 January 2011 < http://journals.humankinetics.com/ijsnem-back-issues/IJSNEM-Volume16Issue1February/ChocolateMilkasaPostExerciseRecoveryAid>.

how much fluid I lost through sweat. I then drink an equal amount, in weight, to replenish what I lost. It is not uncommon to lose anywhere from two to five pounds or more during a really intense wrestling practice, and as you can imagine it is often difficult to down half a gallon of water quick enough to rehydrate. That is where chocolate milk or other recovery drinks come in handy. I have found that it is easier for me to drink more when I enjoy the drink, rather than just plain water. I subtract the amount of chocolate milk from what weight I lost, and that is how much water I drink in addition to the chocolate milk. Unless you want to feel awful, don't chug it all in a matter of minutes. I usually consume the recovery drink pretty fast, but gradually sip the rest of the water over the course of about forty-five minutes. Plus, the sodium and potassium in chocolate milk will aid in replacing lost electrolytes, just as in sports drinks.

5. **Be size wise** – This can get somewhat subjective, so it is important that you accurately and honestly assess your workout. If I just finished a grueling wrestling practice, I usually drink sixteen ounces of chocolate milk. My strength training or conditioning sessions, although tough, aren't as demanding as wrestling, so I generally just have eight ounces after those workouts. The amount of carbohydrates you need will depend largely on how intense the workout was and how big you are. Heavier athletes can probably get away with sixteen ounces after any workout, but someone lighter should stick with just eight. If you are sneaking in some guilt-free dessert instead of liquid, two medium sized cookies is

roughly the right size.

6. **Solid meal an hour later** – After having my
    recovery drink or meal immediately following
    my workout, I usually eat a balanced meal about
    one to one-and-a-half hours after the workout
    ends. By balanced, I mean sensible portions of
    lean proteins, vegetables, and good carbs. As I
    mentioned in point one, you probably don't have
    time to shower, change, and drive home before
    that twenty minute window is up, so not only is a
    recovery drink a nutritionally sound decision, but
    it is a very practical one, too. Instead of rushing
    through my shower and trying to throw a healthy
    meal together in twenty minutes, I consume my
    chocolate milk right after my workout, leaving me
    an hour to stretch (I strongly advise stretching *after*
    a workout), shower, rehydrate, and prepare a meal.

There are however, situations where you won't be able to
follow this plan exactly. For instance, if you are at a relative's house for Thanksgiving and they offer some pumpkin
pie, it would be quite rude to leave your host and say: "Sorry,
I have to work out *right now*! I'll be back in thirty minutes."
If you absolutely can't squeeze in a workout before having dessert, then politely take a moderate portion and savor
it. Oftentimes, a sliver of pie or cake or a single cookie is
enough to satisfy any cravings. It may be hard to stop after
just one helping, but if you've been following these direc-
tions and having chocolate milk or a small dessert after each
workout, chances are you won't feel deprived or have intense cravings. Just enjoy it and get right back on track next
time you work out.

ABOUT JEFF

Jeff Streu is currently a senior electrical engineering student at Rensselaer Polytechnic Institute (RPI) in Troy, NY.

He has been wrestling for nine years and fitness and nutrition have been his passion since then. At RPI he is a captain of the wrestling team and is a two-time NCWA National Qualifier.

Before college he grew up in Arlington Heights, IL, where he attended Buffalo Grove High School. While in high school he was a member of the 2006 and 2007 Team Illinois National Team in both Freestyle and Greco-Roman wrestling.

CHAPTER 11

BE HONEST WITH YOURSELF

BY MIKE SBONIK & JEFF TARDIFF

There are many myths and a lot of mystical answers in the fitness field today when it comes to fat burning and muscle building. Building muscle and burning fat is not as complicated as mainstream sources want you to believe. There are no secrets or anything mysterious about it. You just need to be ready to follow this one simple concept – *Be honest with yourself.* Be willing to step outside yourself and look at the way you are working out and what you are putting into your body. Then ask yourself how this is working for your goal.

I want to get two things straight right from the start. **Diet** is a word that means what we eat on a regular basis, not something that you do temporarily for a result that will only last for a short period of time. "Diets" that only last for a short term will end up making you gain weight in the long run –

once you come off of that diet. Then, the next time you decide to "diet" for a special occasion, you have almost twice as much weight to work off as you did the first time.

The second thing that seems hard for people to understand is that we <u>cannot</u> spot reduce! We burn fat from all over our body and the muscles that we work get toned and harden from building muscle in those areas – such as that person we all know that is losing weight, but not showing any muscle tone in the areas that they want to "shape". There is no tone because they are not building the muscle in that area of their body while they are losing the weight. Thus, frustration comes from people like this who are always trying the latest fad diets, TV gadgets or mystical "no effort" ways, and still not seeing the results they want. We need to start thinking about the results that we want, and then how our workout and eating habits are contributing toward that goal.

If you are trying to build muscle and burn fat, you should not be doing exercises that are meant for strength training or different types of sports performance. How much load are you using? How long are the breaks you are taking? What type of exercises are you doing? Now, more importantly, why? Most people are still following workouts based upon methods that were developed 40 years ago. We just learned about how motor units within the muscles work within the past ten years.

Now we need to look at nutrition with that same mindset. Many people think that if they exercise they can eat whatever they want. Really? Well, I'm here to tell you that about 80% of our fitness results come from what we put into our mouths. There is no secret to it. If you eat **real** food (get the full story on nutrition in our Free Bonus Report) in realistic portions and for the purpose of what you need to do in your day, you will see the results that you work so hard for will be lasting, while you are still enjoying what you eat. I won't lie to you, this takes work. It comes from educating ourselves, discovering how our body works, and a lot of discipline over time. The results that you want that will last a lifetime come with these things. It's easy to follow this system if you stay honest with yourself.

Our body uses specific energy systems at specifics moments in exercise. It is important to understand what energy system we are relying on the most during our workouts, so that our workouts are tailored for our specific goal. For this writing, the goal is burning fat. So it only makes sense to train in the heart rate zone in which you are using more fat as fuel. You'll have to excuse me for getting technical for a minute here. I am not going to get into much depth about it, but I want you to understand more about how our body uses fat as fuel when we exercise.

The body uses adenosine triphosphate (ATP) as energy to contract and relax muscles. In the first 2 – 15 seconds of work, the body is relying mainly on ATP alone to fuel the muscles. After that, the body has to rely on other fuel sources in order to create more ATP for the muscle contractions to happen. The body then relies on the second energy system, which is the glycolytic system. This is the breaking down of glucose and glycogen in order to create more ATP. Glucose is the sugar that is in your blood, while glycogen is stored in the liver and is broken down into glucose, as the body needs it. This energy system is used for up to 2 minutes of highly intense exercise.

The third and final energy system is the oxidative system. Though this system is quite complicated it can simply be described as the body using carbohydrates and fats as long term energy in the presence of oxygen. In fact, fat is our primary source of energy at rest. Using this process, about 1500 calories can be used from carbohydrate energy and 70,000 calories can be used from the breaking down of fat. So as you can see, fat is a better energy source than carbohydrates for a long duration of exercise. The reason our body uses carbohydrates as energy first is because they are easier to break down and take less time to break down into energy that is ready to be used.

Now we can take the above information and look at how our workout relates to the use of these energy systems. If our primary goal is to burn fat, then our workout should be based upon utilizing fat as the primary energy source. How do we go about doing that? Though we never utilize only one of these systems at a time, we can focus more on using our fat as the primary energy source by exercising at about 50% – 70% maximal heart rate for a longer period of time.

If you don't have that kind of time to exercise, this may be hard to do. You may then want to focus on burning the most possible calories within the session. Even though you may not be focusing on the use of fat as the primary energy source by burning as many calories as possible, you keep your body from storing this extra energy, which would eventually be converted into fat.

My personal preference after warming up is to start out at a high intensity level to call upon all three systems as the primary source over the course of my exercise bout. This way, in the beginning I am using up my glucose and glycogen stores and then my body will primarily oxidize carbohydrate energy. Then in order to continue the bout, my body would start to use my fat stores as it's primary energy source. An example of this would be running at as high an intensity level as you can, while continuing to run at that pace for as long as possible.

When you cannot hold that higher intensity any longer, continue to run at a lower intensity level for a long period of time. For most, this would be about 45 minutes or more.

Another great way to utilize all of these systems as the primary energy source is through exercising in intervals. This means you would exercise at a high level of intensity for a short period of time and then bring it to a low intensity for a while, and then another brief period at a high intensity level before bringing it back down to a lower intensity level. This cycle would continue throughout the entire exercise bout.

It is important to understand that this does not apply to only doing aerobic-style workouts. This can also be applied to weight/resistance training. First we must understand the importance of resistance training. Resistance training is geared toward muscle building. Muscle produces heat and burns fat. Even when we are stationary, one pound of muscle added to the body will burn another 50 calories a day.

*Know this, muscle does NOT turn into fat and fat does NOT develop into muscle. They are two completely different types of tissue within the body.

Resistance also builds stronger and thicker bones, which is very important to our long term health as we grow older and our bodies start to develop osteoporosis. Osteoporosis is the process of the bones losing mass and strength. Osteoporosis can even be reversed in the elderly that are utilizing resistance training that is proper for them. So, even women need to utilize resistance training in order to build muscle that is going to burn fat while providing a healthy and toned look to the body, and also building stronger bones. Don't worry, I am not talking about building huge body builder muscles and bones thick enough to make you seem wider. I am talking about the muscle and bone structure that you need to develop in order to reach your goals more effectively, maintain these results for life, and to do it in a healthy manner.

Let's know now that as far as whether training muscle endurance, muscle strength or for muscle hypertrophy (building in size), all of these are going to develop muscle that is going to help my body burn fat. The difference is at which level each one is helping toward the goal. The first step is to have an understanding of each one. I can't even begin to tell you how many people I see doing different kinds of resistance exercises that aren't even geared toward their goal. So here is a brief outline of how this works without going too far in depth.

Muscle endurance – a lower weight for a high amount of repetitions (at least more then 12) with less then a 30 second break between sets. This is not limited to repetitions; you can even lift the weight for a timed period such as a minute straight or even 5 minutes straight. This is going to build muscles that are smaller in size, but can handle the task at hand for a longer period of time. Depending on the system you use, you will only want to do 2 – 3 sets if you are counting the amount of reps or a short period of time, such as a minute. Do only one set if you were lifting the weight for 4 – 5 minutes straight.

Muscle hypertrophy (building muscles that are larger in mass) – a high amount of weight for 6 – 12 repetitions with only 30 – 90 second breaks. Your weight should be at a level in which the muscles feel exhausted after each set. This should be applied for 3 – 6 sets. This will build muscles that are larger in mass. This can be applied without exhausting the muscle in every set, however, the reason I say to do so is so that you also gain more muscle strength and endurance in the process.

<u>Muscle Strength/Power</u> – a very high amount of weight for only 6 repetitions or less with a 2 – 5 minute break between sets. The muscle should not be exhausted in this type of workout. Every repetition should have the same amount of effort involved. The repetitions should be performed in an explosive type manner, which means you let the weight drop quickly, and with no pause at the bottom of the rep, lift the weight as quickly as possible. The point behind this type of training is NOT to build muscle mass. It is used to build muscle strength through the building of motor units within the muscle. This basically works by building the ability to call more muscle strands into action at one given moment.

This is important to know so we can look at how effective our workout is for reaching our goal. So now we know that if I want to build muscle, I should not take two-minute breaks or more in-between sets. We also know now that there is a big difference between strength training and muscle building, along with the fact that muscle mass does not always mean strength. This is an important point because so many people, especially guys, think that they have to put on a large amount of mass in order to be stronger and this is simply not true. Mass may provide more power through inertia, but actual muscle strength and power will come from the ability to call more motor units into action at one time. It also important to note that the growth of muscle mass will also depend primarily upon calorie and protein intake.

So what is the most effective method for toning up and burning fat? Muscle building along with muscle endurance training will be the most effective for this goal along with some type of aerobic training along with it. Basically the muscle will be burning fat while aerobic work is burning the extra calories that your body does not need for your regular daily functioning. By doing the aerobics, not only are you working the cardiovascular system, but you are also getting rid of the extra carbohydrates to keep them from being converted into stored energy such as fat, while burning off the fat that is already there.

Following are three workout routines that have demonstrated results. The first is an example of a 'dumbbell circuit' workout that is geared toward building muscle and burning fat. You can do this at home with two dumbbells. I highly suggest starting light and less than the suggested repetitions until you know that you are able to do this. Once you are able to do this workout and it is getting easier, go to doing three sets of each exercise. The reason we start with three sets in the lower body exercises right away is to build the large muscle groups of the lower body because we burn twice as many calories when we do so. Go through this workout with no breaks. This workout should take no more than an hour.

	Dynamic Stretches	10 Min. Jump Rope	
2 sets	15 – 20 Push ups	15 – 20 crunches	
2 sets	10 – 12 Single arm Bicep Curls	10 – 12 Overhead Triceps Extensions	15 – 20 Leg Raises
2 sets	10 – 12 Upright Rows	10 – 12 Overhead Press	15 – 20 Back Extensions
2 sets	8 – 10 Lateral Raises	8 – 10 Front Shoulder Raises	40 Flutter Kicks
3 sets	10 – 12 Lunges	10 – 12 Diamond Push ups	
2 sets	25 – 30 Shoulder Shrugs	1 Min. Plank	
2 sets	10 – 12 Bent Over Rows	10 Slow Alternating Oblique Twists While laying Down	
2 sets	10 – 12 Two Arm Bicep Curls	10 ea. Side Sitting Oblique Twists With a Ball or Small Dumbbell in Hand	
3 sets	12 Squats	10 ea. Leg Single leg Lifts While Standing	
3 sets	15 – 20 Calve Raises	15 – 20 Wide Hand Push Up	
	Cool Down	Static Stretches	

The second is a 'reverse pyramid' workout that is also geared toward muscle building/fat burning. For this workout you will start off each exercise with a weight that only allows you to do 4 – 5 reps. Each set after that, take off 10 – 15% of the weight and do as many repetitions as you can until failure. Repeat this step for three or more sets with only 30 – 60 second breaks in between sets. Do this with the following exercises. Feel free to add in more exercises if you wish, but make sure you are doing all of these first.

Bench Press
Squats
Rows
Lunges
Bicep Curls
Triceps Extension
Calve Raises
Lateral Shoulder Raises
Front Shoulder Raises
Crunches
Back Extensions

*Do not go as heavy on the crunches and back extensions.

The third is a workout for muscle building. Take no more than 30 – 60 second breaks between each set.

	Dynamic Stretches	Warm Up
Bench Press	4 – 5 sets	8 – 12 reps
Squats	4 – 5 sets	8 – 12 reps
Two Arm Bicep Curls	4 – 5 sets	8 – 12 reps
Two Armed Triceps Extension	4 – 5 sets	8 – 12 reps
Lunges	4 – 5 sets	8 – 12 reps
Rows	4 – 5 sets	8 – 12 reps
Leg Extensions	4 – 5 sets	8 – 12 reps
Lateral Shoulder Raise	4 – 5 sets	8 – 12 reps
Leg Curl	4 – 5 sets	8 – 12 reps

Front Shoulder Raise	4 – 5 sets	8 – 12 reps
Calve Raises	4 – 5 sets	8 – 12 reps
Single Arm Bicep Curls	4 – 5 sets	8 – 12 reps
Single Arm Triceps Extension	4 – 5 sets	8 – 12 reps
Crunches w/weight	4 – 5 sets	8 – 12 reps
Back Extensions	4 – 5 sets	8 – 12 reps
	Cool Down	Static Stretches

[*I suggest you get assessed by a trainer or physician before participating in any of the above workouts. I also suggest yoga for flexibility training. That is a good example of a workout in which you are utilizing your fat for energy almost the entire time.]

The more important question when thinking about fat burning and muscle building is, what do we put into our bodies? Remember, we are no longer thinking with the mindset that exercise is the complete answer to losing weight and getting toned. Start thinking in the manner that 80% of the results you get will come from what you eat.

First of all, the most important part of real health and maintaining a healthy body with the results throughout our lifetime is eating real food. Stop confusing your body with fad diets or 'yo-yoing'. Believe me, you are just making the problem worse. Be consistent with how much you are eating on a daily basis and eat real food. (Get the full story on nutrition in our Free Bonus Report.)

Building muscle and burning fat is not as difficult as it may seem. You have to learn to *be honest with yourself*. Ask yourself the following questions: Is this work out geared toward my goal? How is what I am about to eat going to help me with what I have to do today? Is it? If not, why are you eating it or doing that workout?

We must also remember that we are human. You will not be perfect. You will fail at making the right decisions from time to time. But guess what? That's okay. It is all a part of learning and getting better at learning about our bodies. The important thing is that we get back on track and keep ourselves focused over the long term, and realize that it is all about discipline over time. You will get better at this and your body will respond. Surround yourself with the lifestyle you want and that's what you'll become.

ABOUT JEFF

Jeff Tardiff has become a sought-out fitness and nutrition consultant because he lives the example of "being true to yourself."

One of his latest examples has been working with his mother to help her lose weight in a healthy manner with no fad diets. Since then, she has lost over 100 pounds and feels 'light-years' better.

Jeff was a competitor in numerous sports and excelled in grappling for over 12 years due to his 'never quit' attitude. After high school, he enlisted in the United States Air Force and earned a spot as a TACP (one of the Air Force special operation jobs).

He was class leader and got perfect scores on every physical fitness test, which is no small feat. Jeff was chosen to go to airborne school, survival school and air assault school. While stationed with the 82nd airborne division at Fort Bragg, he was able to train in modern combat.

After leaving the military, Jeff received his diploma from Penn Foster Career School as a Fitness/Nutritionist. Jeff is MAT Jumpstart Certified and also holds a Resistance Training Specialist designation. He is enrolled at Globe University in the Health and Fitness Specialist program for the Bachelor of Science degree.

Jeff is a top black belt trainer in Kung Ling Kung Fu™, where he was chosen to represent this reality self-defense system to the world and is a top fitness trainer for the local YMCA.

Jeff Tardiff believes in natural longevity through proper fitness and eating real food. He coaches people everyday how to achieve their best.

To learn more about Jeff Tardiff and how you can receive free fitness reports visit the exclusive kung fu site: www.kunglingkungfu.com and sign up for the free Master Tips e-newletter today.

ABOUT MIKE

Mike Sbonik is known as a "fitness aficionado." He's the guy that demonstrates that you can look and feel half your age.

Mike spent his formative years working on the family farm in WI where he experienced first-hand the Midwest work ethic.

Since he weighed less than 100 pounds in high school, he found his niche in wrestling and cross-country running, and found that competition drove Mike to "always do the best you can."

He pursued his dream of being a martial artist in college. Then over the span of 20 years learned many martial arts systems to round out his combat experience; Tae Kwon Do, Pa Kua Chung kung fu, Hwa Rung Do, Brazilian Jiu Jitsu, American boxing, Muy Thai kickboxing, Lima Lama, and Eskrima.

His Muy Thai experience culminated in a modified rules match at the age of 39 when his opponent was 22. Mike focuses on proper working out methods, especially the 'as you age' philosophy, and you can still find him competing in local 5k races.

Mike is a top black belt trainer in Kung Ling Kung Fu™, where he was chosen to represent this reality self-defense system to the world and is a volunteer board member for the local YMCA where he can be found living his "fitness aficionado" lifestyle.

Mike Sbonik's training techniques are all about natural strength and endurance fitness, by working out to be able to protect your family at any moment. He lives this philosophy every day.

To learn more about Mike Sbonik and how you can receive free fitness reports, visit the exclusive kung fu site: www.kunglingkungfu.com and sign up for free Master Tips e-newsletter today.

CHAPTER 12

WEIGHT LOSS CONFUSION IN AMERICA, ONE MAN'S PERSPECTIVE

BY MIKE STARKS

In the fall of 2005, life was good (or so I thought). I had sold my company the previous year and was able to 'retire'. No worries, no stress, another daughter in my family. Things were just grand until….

There are moments in a man's life where he knows and understands just how stupid the look of a woman can make him feel. It was one of those looks from my wife that changed my life. I was sitting on our bed watching college football and enjoying my stress-free life. My wife ran into the bedroom and was going to meet some girlfriends to do those 'girlfriend things'. As she was changing her shirt I glanced over and noticed she had on her $300 overpriced Trendy Woman maternity pants. You know the ones that look super sexy from the waist down but like a diaper with elastic from the waist up. (Now, this is a man's opinion. We of course have no design sense, so there's no need to get offended). When my wife makes fun of my man things (tools, sports, etc.), I simply realize she has no clue about my 'man thing world' and therefore I just smile and nod my head. Now back to the pants. So casually (and cordially) I asked, "Honey, why are you still wearing your maternity pants?" And then it occurred. The 'look'! The look that screams 'You Idiot. You clueless idiot who can't straighten your sock drawer without calling your mother.' You know the 'look'. It also doubles as the look of death.

I knew immediately I was in trouble. I had only experienced this 'look' a few times in my life. My mom gave me the look when she bailed me out of jail once. My high school girlfriend gave me the look when I told a waiter on our prom that "She needs more time to look at the menu cause she's on a diet." Yes…every man knows the look. Even scarier, every woman knows the look and how to 'dish out' the look at the speed of light. The look takes no prisoners. It is simply meant to destroy all dumbfounded men in its path. As the father of three young daughters, I can testify that women learn the look the moment they are conceived. My daughters give me the look several times a day and it scares the 'bejesus' out of me.

So there was the look. I knew immediately I had crossed the line. I had killed the first born. I had done something yet I had no clue what I had done. The deep meaningful words that followed out of my mouth often takes a man years to perfect, "What, what did I say?"

The words that followed were pushed out by some demon. It was as if my lips wanted to say "You are the prettiest woman I have ever seen." Yet these life-changing words came out instead…"It's been 6 months since you had the baby why are you still wearing maternity pants?" There, I said it. I did not mean to say it but I said it. Seconds seemed like days as 'the look' was closing in for the kill.

Amazingly enough my wife looked at me and patiently responded "I can't lose weight like I used to…it's getting harder and harder." Then she finished buttoning her top, which covered the diaper elastic portion of her $300 maternity pants, ran out of the bedroom and left me in a bewildered state between college football and a near-death experience.

While my wife was gone that day, I decided in order to make up my for my stupid man comment, I would need to show her that with diaper pants and all that I still loved her. This was my chance to 'help' her lose weight and get back into those size ?? pants. (Ladies, men do not know nor will they ever understand your sizing. With 2's, 4's, etc. you may as well use planet names like, 'I wear size Uranus', …we just don't get it.)

Upon my wife's return from her girls night out 'thing', I was excitedly waiting like a puppy dog. I had come up with a solution to her dilemma. I knew she would go for it because it meant that I would do all the cooking and cleaning. My wife is a 90's woman. Never has cooked, most likely never will. We had a full-time cook while I was working but she passed away shortly after I sold my business, and therefore my wife had resorted to other means of eating.

So, when my wife walked in that night, I immediately began to tell her my game plan like a coach in a locker room. Very cautiously, I informed her about my observations on why she could not lose the 'after-baby fat'. I told her that because God gave her such a big heart she always put her family and friends in front of herself. Now I really did not believe this, but I was in apology mode. And when a man is in apology mode, he does unthinkable things that he will not even admit to his man friends. Anyway, I told her because she was always tending to others she simply had no time to take care of herself. She would skip meals and then munch on junk all day. …Eating a raisin here, …some trail mix there. …A cup of yogurt or a sandwich with organic honey and peanut butter with wholewheat crackers, etc. So, throughout the day she would snack. Then at night, in her head, with the speed and accuracy of a 10 key, she would add up the calories and determine how many she had left for the day. Within the blink of an eye she would head into the kitchen and party like a rock star on cake, wine and anything else as long as it kept her under her total calories.

So I made a deal with my wife. I would cook her simple meats and vegetables, freeze them in a bag every Sunday night so all she had to do throughout her multi-tasking week was grab a meat and vegetable, nuke it for a minute and get on with life. She agreed. More importantly, she forgave me for my man comment!

Five months later and 55 lbs less, my wife happily ebay'ed her maternity pants and strutted around in life like a new-found woman. Her confidence was scary. Her self-esteem was through the roof. We were both amazed that by simply eating old-fashioned foods like meats, vegetables and eggs, that she could lose so much weight without killing herself in the gym. Could it be this simple? Just eat old fashioned natural foods without all the processed carbs and sugars?

Thinking this may be an anomaly, I decided to test out my theory of weight loss simplicity on a group of teachers. Fifteen teachers at a school volunteered to take the challenge and eat this way for six weeks if I provided the food for free.

The results? In 6 weeks, all 15 teachers lost between 13 and 24 lbs. by simply eating natural foods and avoiding sugar, processed carbohydrates, certain dairy and nut fats.

With this group of teachers we learned some very simple and practical rules for success in dieting...

1. Food must taste good
2. Plan must require hardly any thinking. Grab it and eat
3. Food must be prepared, eaten and cleaned up in minutes
4. Food cannot contain processed fillers like rice, pasta, gravies, etc.
5. Food must have variety
6. Food must be filling
7. The whole concept must be simple to understand, implement and manage
8. Accountability increases odds of success
9. Starving yourself cannot be part of the plan
10. Exercising <u>more</u> is often a detriment because it fools you into believing you can eat anything you want
11. Food must be affordable

If you are like me, I cannot stand studies. There are studies that support just about anything you can think of. With that being said, I was not satisfied with my newfound study. Forgiven by my wife but still restless, I wanted to know. I wanted to understand why America was doing the exact opposite of what just worked for my wife and this group of teachers. We were being told to count calories, avoid fat, exercise hard, starve if you have to, and be mentally tough.

As I dove into the depths of Google and into the dark side of the fat man's curse, I began seeing a pattern that was plain as day. Now again, I was not biased at the time. I had nothing to gain or lose. I simply had to know why something so obvious was so overlooked.

Before I share this new found pattern, let me say I believe the best and most accurate assessments on obesity are not studies, clinics or experiments. The best 'proven' study in the world is simply facts based on historical civilizations. Follow their trend long enough and you discover their habits, which affect millions of people.

I am a huge believer in Occam's Razor... "the simplest path is often the best path." In America, as you will discover below, we have made weight loss and fitness a rather complex and convoluted process. Our weight loss theory is far from simple and has resulted in complete failure. Again, this is not an opinion, this is fact. Could it be possible that all the experts and their studies are missing the mark? Think about it... America is the most obese country in the world and, oddly enough, the most nutritionally educated country in the history of the world. Respectfully I ask again, "Are we doing something wrong?"

Have entire civilizations missed the mark before? Have they followed a path of destruction for several years then finally realized their theory or beliefs were simply wrong? You bet they have. Today I present to you one of these misdiagnoses in America that changed the course of our medical community and the health of the American people in more ways than one. Smoking.

I recall growing up with parents who smoked. Most of their

friends smoked. Most of our neighbors smoked. Most doctors smoked. The old TV shows from the 1950's show doctors in a hospital reviewing a patient's chart while most of them were dragging away on a cancer stick. Amazingly, the medical community agreed that smoking was harmless. Study after study proved that smoking had no serious effects on health. All of this overwhelming proof yet Lung Cancer and Heart Disease were soaring in America. Look at the chart below (figure 1) and you will see the rate of increase among smokers in the USA along with heart disease and Lung Cancer. It's as plain as day, yet we ignored the signs, because the 'experts' and the government had convinced us that smoking was safe.

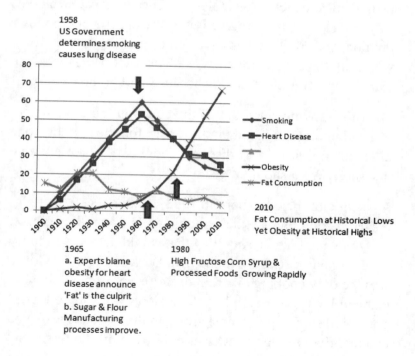

1965 –
THE BEGINNING OF OBESITY IN AMERICA

Now, this is my belief or theory, it is not a fact but if you look at the correlation between the two I believe you will see what I base my observations on. In 1960, obesity in America was scarce. However heart disease was at an all-time high. The government could not figure out why so many people were dying of heart attacks. Smoking was ruled out because all the tests and studies had proven that smoking was not harmful. There were a few studies which showed contradicting results but the 'experts' and medical community considered them cynical quacks. Again, let me repeat this yet in another way… "Those who disagreed with the experts and popular opinion were ridiculed and labeled as cynical idiots." Even worse, all the experts (doctors, scientists, etc.) supported the 'Smoking is Harmless' theory because a lot of them smoked!

So with smoking ruled out of the equation the government began looking for another diagnosis for the number one killer in America, heart disease. They had to take extreme measures. What should they do?

As a child of the 60's (born in 1963), I often recall the Folgers can sitting on our kitchen counter. It was full of grease, lard, cooking oil, etc. Anything that would help my mom fry food without it sticking to the pan. Back in the 60's, Crisco was the only cooking oil around. Bottles of Canola oil, vegetable oil, etc. were simply non-existent. Why buy oil when you could simply get your share from the various meats you cooked. Everything we ate was cooked in oil. I still see my Mom digging a big spoon into the hardened lard and slapping it in the skillet. Every household in America ate this way. Now remember, America did not have an obesity issue

WEIGHT LOSS CONFUSION IN AMERICA, ONE MAN'S PERSPECTIVE

back in 1965 or prior. Even though we ate lots of fat, lard, oil, meat, etc. Could this be the answer? Was fat consumption increasing right along with Heart and Lung disease? Interestingly enough the answer is a simple 'No'. For the past several hundred years, society has used animal fat for cooking food. It had not increased or decreased and yet it now had just become America's #1 Killer – the demon of heart disease.

With fat now in their crosshairs, the experts and US government felt like they had enough solid evidence to put their newfound theory on trial. To support their case they began study after study which led us to believe that the consumption of fat was the true culprit in heart disease. Said another way, "They believed people were having heart attacks because they were consuming too much fat." Notice I did not say 'Food', I said 'Fat'. Sometime around 1965, the government began developing the infamous food pyramid. I recall it well. There were certain variations of it because the government refused to create the actual graphic. They left this up to various educational systems to create their own graphic interpretation. In 1968 during my first year in kindergarten, I recall being forced to learn a food pyramid and all the food groups. Of course I ignored it because the only food I cared about was candy. Interesting enough, candy or sugar was not on a lot of the food pyramid charts back then. They did not say it was good or bad. So, like most kids, I assumed it could not be that bad if they made no mention of it.

So, our problems seem to be solved. Fat was indicted and given a life sentence. It was Fat responsible for killing everyone so all the experts now began telling us to avoid Fat. Being the herd we are, we listened and since their sermons of the 60's began, we have paid the price dearly.

HOW AND WHY AMERICA GOT FAT...

As I began my research, I quickly realized there was no government or hidden corporate conspiring body out to 'make America Fat' or to mislead Americans. It simply happened over a period of time. Some misunderstandings, a few large corporations (persuasive of course) and some biased studies have led to popular belief and conventional wisdom. Unfortunately when corporations began seeing the profits of this newfound fat theory, our course of disorientation went into extreme fat man vertigo. We were getting fatter and so was their balance sheet. Over the past 40 years, many companies have seen record

revenues based on a misunderstanding of obesity. But hey, that's capitalism at the cost of a culture. No hard feelings, it's just business.

Okay, so let's look at the facts. For the past 45 years since 1965....

1. Fat consumption has declined
2. Calorie consumption has slightly increased by about 5%
3. Obesity has skyrocketed from 6% of the American population in 1965 to about 65% in 2010.

So has fat consumption and eating too much made us fat? Obviously not. So what has? What are we doing differently today than we did 45 years ago? Now, before you spit out the patented 'We are less active' answer, I want to respectfully challenge this conventional wisdom with this fact. Japanese children are less active than American children. They go to 2 schools, primary in the day, secondary in the night. They play more video games per capita than American kids do...

meaning they are much less active than our kids. Yet the Japanese do not have an obesity issue. So what is it?

More facts…

1. The **manufacturing process of sugar & flour has improved tremendously**
2. The **consumption of sugar has skyrocketed**
3. The **consumption of flour has skyrocketed**

And even more facts…

1. Countries that **consume excessive sugar and processed carbohydrates are ALL obese** and suffer from type 2 diabetes, hypertension, syndrome X, etc.
2. Countries that **avoid sugar and processed carbohydrates** and yet **consume natural foods like meats, vegetables, nuts, select dairy** products tend to be very healthy with very little disease and very little obesity issues.
3. Countries that **avoid sugar and processed carbohydrates** and **yet consume animal fats (yes, even saturated fats)** tend to be very healthy with very little disease and very little obesity issues.

Now before you set this book down, run out and buy meats and veggies, and torment your family with another diet (trust me, your family is tormented every time you mention the 'D' word), I highly recommend you understand all the elements of weight loss: your body, why we are fat, how we became fat and why we, the most nutritionally-educated civilization in the history of the world (the United States), are backwards in our weight loss attempts.

What I am about to tell you is difficult for most people in

America to believe because it has been conventional wisdom for the past 40 years. It has been so ingrained in our heads that we consider it almost a sacred religion. A religion that 90% of the US population follow with the conviction of a martyr.

Fat and calories do not create body fat!

There I said it. Classify me as another quack. Facebook or Twitter that Mike Starks is a rule breaker who hates authority (okay, in a way I do). That the CEO of The Meal Movement has no clue what he is talking about. (*Favor: If you choose to post crazy things about me, all I ask is that you put a picture of Brad Pitt by my name. People may dislike the things I say but at least they will have a good mental image of me!)

Interestingly enough, in the 70's, many biochemistry experiments (facts not opinions) proved that consumption of fat cannot create fat cells. It simply could not happen. Eat fat on bacon and it cannot create body fat. It's like saying if you drink a coke, your skin will turn brown. Meat fat cannot create fat. Yet these 'proven' biochemistry experiments were overlooked because they were not accepted by the experts and they went against what the experts and the government were preaching. The experiments surely must be wrong.

So in the late 70's while America began decreasing their consumption of fat ...obesity continued its assault on America. Next, the experts turned to 'caloric theory'. Caloric theory is simply the measurement of heat exchange. It was created by Clement in 1824 for the measurement of steam. Since then it has been used in the nutritional world because of one thing...it has made a lot of corporations billions of dollars. Companies build and brand entire lines of food based on 'low calorie' labels. Their formula works like this:

Great Taste + Low Calorie = Lots of money

Don't believe me? Look at Nabisco's 100 Calorie packs.

So why do we buy the low fat, low calorie theory? Because it's easy to visualize and to understand very quickly. Close your eyes and think about eating a large steak with some fat on it. See the meat and fat going into your stomach then being converted into fat on your butt or thighs? Or see the fat going into your blood stream and creating blood clots. It's very easy to conceptualize therefore its believable and an easy sale. So what about calories? Caloric theory goes something like this ...Eat more than you exert and you gain weight, eat less than you exert and you lose weight. Again it's an easy to understand model that we can quickly analyze and say... 'makes sense to me!!!'

MYTH OF THE FLAT EARTH

From 330 AD up to the 17th century, most countries believed the earth was flat. Before you comment on how ridiculous this sounds, you must understand that countries and entire civilizations believed this because all the experts and governments agreed in this theory. Galileo was sent to the inquisition for affirming that the earth was a sphere. Those who disagreed with the 'experts' and their conventional wisdom were steamrolled and classified as cynical quacks. The lesson here? That governments and experts are infallible too. That their studies, experiments, research, etc. can contain error. Again, we believed smoking was okay from 1900 to 1960. Even after Germany began linking smoking to lung cancer in 1920, we simply discredited 'those Nazi criminals' because we did not like them.

THE TRUE CULPRIT(S)

I remember taking a helicopter tour in Hawaii and the pilot pointing to the closed sugar cane plantations. He informed us that it took something like 50 tons of water to produce 1 pound of sugar. Before 1960 sugar manufacturing was a tedious and costly endeavor. Since then, the manufacturing process has become very efficient and with the birth of High Fructose corn syrup, sweetening food is as easy as pie. Same thing with the flour industry. In 1960 the average American ate around 60 pounds of sugar a year. Today the average American eats over 165 lbs of sugar a year. So is the correlation between sugar and obesity a coincidence? I don't think so.

Again, look at civilizations and their trends. With a little re-search you will find that ALL (yes ALL), countries who eat excessive sugar or flour products suffer from obesity, type 2 diabetes, syndrome X, increased cancer rates, etc. While those who eat meats (and meat fat), vegetables, eggs and nuts do not.

So where do fruits and whole grains fit in? I was afraid you were going to ask that…classify me as a quack (again). Civili-zations who ate lots of whole grain products and fruit suffered from similar obesity, diseases, etc., similar to those who ate lots of sugar. The old Egyptians are a classic example.

Hey, don't kill the messenger. I am just providing facts. Sim-ply Google 'Obesity Epidemic in Pacific Islands.' Here's a country that prior to 1940 had some of the healthiest people in the world. Their islands were a stopping point for a lot of the American troops and their diets went from fish, island animals, local fruits and vegetables to sugar, flour, white rice, canned fruits, soft drinks and beer. Their obesity rates are now as high as 75% and they have children at the age of ten being diagnosed with type 2 diabetes (type 1 is juvenile diabetes, while type 2 is self-induced and occurs from wearing the body out by too much glucose spiking or obesity).

There, I said it. I got it off my chest. Call me a cynical quack or call me genius. I just know at the age of 48 I simply avoid processed carbs, sugar and some dairy fat.

I have great health (for now!) and I don't see any old man diaper elastic pants in my future!

My hope for all who read this chapter is that it makes sense. Sense enough that you, your spouse or your clients will get to experience the weight loss and healthy lifestyle which can be achieved by simply eating meats, vegetables, eggs, some dairy fat items and select nuts. And that you will be able to ignore most of the complex conventional wisdom long enough to experience the 'aha' moment.

Many humble thanks for sticking with me and reading my chapter.

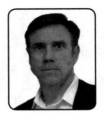

ABOUT MIKE

Mike Starks is the founder, CEO & President of The Meal Movement and Personal Trainer Food – weight loss diet-meal delivery programs. He enjoys working with his passion, weight loss.

Mike started and built six companies with his last two being extremely successful, reaching $30 million in sales. He sold his last company in 2004, and accidentally discovered the keys to weight loss while losing a lot of money in the stock market.

"It was an expensive lesson but well worth it!" says Starks.

He's very passionate about weight loss through eating right and not so much about laborious exercise. He should know, at 48 years old Mike Starks is very proud of maintaining 6-7% body fat by simply walking 30 minutes a day and eating the right foods.

"My goal is to see America get back to the basics of eating. To forget all this rocket science nutrition and workout methodology stuff. It's simple... just eat Meats, Vegetables, Natural Dairy and you get to your ideal weight. No need for seaweed, kelp or organic meatballs. Just simple old-fashioned foods like we ate 50 years ago without all the processed stuff. This is my passion, to educate people back to simplicity (and hopefully make a little money while doing it!)."

He enjoys playing tag and frisbee with his children during his off time. He also has a heart for troubled and abused kids who just need a break and a little bit of direction.

"I used to hunt, fish and travel; buy goofy things like cars, planes, boats, etc. Now I am grown up. I like the simpler things in life like family, work and simplicity! I do have a heart for troubled kids. The biggest crime they have committed is being born into their lousy world. We are responsible to help these kids."

Mike lives in Highland Village, Texas with his wife and three daughters.

CHAPTER 13

FOUR SIMPLE STEPS TO WORLD DOMINATION...FOR WOMEN...

BY DR. JENNIFER RADA, D.C.

Hello Ladies! I'm going to give you all of my knowledge and share with you my 4 Simple Steps to World Domination for Women! My big promise to you is this: "If you follow the 4 simple steps in this chapter – you won't be able to stop the sexy-train that is coming your way! If you take my advice and apply it, I promise: you will be leaner, more toned, have more energy and you will rule your world!"

Yes, these are pretty big promises! We can do it! But before I share the magic formula to guaranteed success, consider the truth in this positive quote:

"Simple, fun steps applied over time create massive change."

Wouldn't you agree? If you are like me, you know things have to be 'simple and fun to get em done!' That's why we are going to look at exercise in a whole new way. Together we are going to say, "No!" to hours of boring treadmill work and half-hearted moving, like lukewarm zombies droning through a line of workout machines! Yuk! No more.

If you're ready for something new and you're ready to bring the *real you* – the powerful, beautiful woman you know you are, then we have been brought together for a reason. I will be your guide and we are going to rock this!

BUT FIRST, WHY SHOULD YOU LISTEN TO ME?

I have been a personal fitness trainer for more than 2 decades. I'm also a doctor of chiropractic and perhaps most importantly, I have been where you are. I have been overweight and out of shape. I overcame this to be a Figure Competition Champion and a finalist in a state qualifying regional body building show! Also, I have worked with a huge variety of training clients:

- Clients who had never lifted a weight in their lives!
- Clients that had been working out for years and wanted to break through to new success!
- One woman was even training for her first physical fitness test for the FBI academy in Quantico Virginia!

Talk about a variety of cases! I'm going to share with you a real life sneak peek into the challenges and successes one of my favorite clients, Beth. Chances are you'll see part of yourself in her story. You can walk with her during the highs & lows of her journey towards world domination!

Here will be the 4 big take-a-ways for you when you fin-

ish reading this chapter:

- ✓ Fat Loss: You can lose weight. Believe it, because it's true. I will show you how!
- ✓ Toned & Beautiful Muscles: You can get lean, tones muscles without looking manly. Just follow my lead.
- ✓ Energized: You can have more energy. All day. Every day.
- ✓ Dominate: You will know how to use your power for good and reach all your goals! Oh yeah baby!

Now, as your coach I say, "It's time! Let's get moving!"

BETH'S STORY:

When I first saw Beth, she was 45 pounds overweight. She had a warm smile and a profound shyness. Beth also had a burning goal to lose weight for a friend's upcoming wedding. She seemed to have everything going for her, although I could tell there was something fueling her desire to overeat. As it turned out, I would have to be patient, because it would be weeks before she was willing to share her *real* story with me!

At our first meeting, we set her goals in writing. Beth wanted to:

- ➢ Lose 20 pounds in three months
- ➢ Gain muscle tone
- ➢ Raise her self-confidence

Wow! Can you imagine how great it will feel when **you** reach your goals? It can be done...read on.

TO DO: Take 5 minutes now and write down your top 3 goals. Post them on your bathroom mirror.

We prioritized Beth's plan and started with the area that would bring the fastest benefits:

STEP #1:
FAT LOSS

We had to get Beth losing some unwanted body fat to start with visible changes. Our goal was to keep it simple! This is what I put together for Beth:

Rule #1: No Fad Diets – Promise me. Promise me, you will STOP trying at the latest fad! One of my favorite quotes about diets:

> Think about it: if you're eating, then you're on a diet. The only question is, "Are you on a *good diet*?"

So what makes up a good diet? Keep It Simple:

1. **Low to No Refined Sugars:** limit sugary foods, candies and four pump venti lattes.
2. **Eat in moderation**: stop eating when you are comfortably full, not stuffed.
3. **Plan what you *are* going to eat:** rather than worrying about what *not* to eat. For example. plan and prepare tomorrow's food, today.
4. **Dress up your water.** I'm floored at how many of my clients say, "I hate water!" I say with love, "How can you hate water? It's 80% of what you're made of?!"

Well if you find yourself in the water-haters group, take heart; I just happen to have some special tips just for you:

- Add a slice of lemon, lime, cucumber (yes, it is good), orange, etc.
- Consider adding a bit of honey and heating up your water
- Add decaffeinated tea

Bottom line is, you need water and you don't get an adequate supply from other drinks. PLUS other drinks add needless calories that you could be investing in eating food!

Rule #2: Slow Cardio is Your Friend – You don't have to kill yourself doing aggressive cardio exercise to burn fat. In fact, lower intensity cardio burns fat better than high intensity!

<u>A recent study proved:</u>

Exercising 3 times/day for 10 minutes each time burns more calories than one 30 minute session a day!

So break it up. Do something fun. It does not have to be on a treadmill at the gym!

Mix it up...

1. Yoga
2. Biking/Hiking/Kayaking
3. Ballroom Dance Classes (Waaay cooler than you might think)
4. Walking your dog (or a humane society dog)
5. Make up something fun on your own...just do it!

When Beth applied these simple changes to Step #1: Fat Loss: she noticed a nice steady loss of body fat, about 1–2 pounds per week. Her confidence was building.

TO DO: Set a goal you can reach. Then set a new one. Calculate how much total fat you would lose if you lost

1-2 pounds per week for 12 weeks. Write it down.

After the first week Beth had her new routine down and we moved into Step #2.

STEP #2:
TONED & BEAUTIFUL MUSCLES

You have heard women say: "I can't lift weights because I don't want to look like a man." Let me start by saying, "I totally understand." We've all

> *Anyone who denies that is flat out lying!*

seen the she-men on television and thought, "I would never want to look like that!" The good news is…you won't! Trust me there are a lot of prescription & non-prescription drugs involved in a woman getting that big. Anyone who denies that is flat-out lying! So let this worry go, ladies. Trust me.

Beth had this same concern. She thought women always stuck to the 'machines' in the gym because otherwise, they would get big muscles. MYTH!

In fact, whole body movements (WBM's), also known as compound joint movements, burn more calories and create better muscle tone than the isolation movements provided by the lifting 'machines' in the gym. Bottom line ladies, you will have better tone, be more slender, and be stronger if you use compound movements over lifting machines.

Here's the initial workout I designed for Beth:

Beth's Workout Routine:

Day 1: Chest	Incline Dumbbell Press	Bench Press	Hindu Push Ups
Day 2: Back	Cable Pull Downs	Dumbbell Rows	Seated Rows

Day 3: Biceps & Shoulders	Seated Dumbbell Press	Incline Dumbbell Press	Dumbbell Curls
Day 4: Triceps & Calves	Overhead Dumbbell Press	Cable Press Downs	Seated Calf Raises
Day 5: Legs	Hindu Squats	Wide Stance Dumbbell Squats	Narrow Stance Dumbbell Squats
Day 6: Cardio & Abs	Something Fun for 30 – 60 minutes	V-ups for Abs	
Day 7: Rest			

Each day included 3 sets of each exercise with 10 reps each. Notice, we included WBM's. Our goal was to activate multiple muscle groups during each movement to maximize the calories burned.

Perceived Exertion: How hard you feel you are working.

Another Key Point to Remember is your exertion level. You can do all of these exercises and never break a sweat if you choose, or you could do them to your maximum effort & risk injuring yourself. So what is best?

Rating	Description	Training Goal
0	Rest	
1	Very, Very Easy	
2	Easy	
3	Moderate	Fat Loss
4	Somewhat Hard	Fat Loss
5	Hard	Fat Loss
6	Hard	Muscle Building
7	Very Hard	Muscle Building
8	Very Hard	Muscle Building
9	Very Hard	
10	Maximum Effort	

Stay in the zone that is appropriate for your goal that day. Example: if you are on a pure cardio day (meaning no weight lifting) then you would work at an exertion level from 3 – 5.

If you are lifting weights, you should warm your muscles up with 10–15 minutes of cardiovascular exercise and then, working with a trainer; strive to get into a perceived exertion level ranging from 6 – 8, as shown on the table above.

Beth and I were now nearly one month into her training and she was rockin' it! She experienced a few down days, but always picked herself up again and got right back on track. With that type of commitment, she was sure to succeed. Beth had been patient, and was finally starting to really feel the third benefit of her work. She said she was experiencing energy levels like she had never known before! (Still no secret revealed though).

TO DO: What P.E. Level do you want to operate in on day #6 in Beth's Routine?

And that is what leads us into Step #3.

STEP #3:
ENERGIZED

We could all use more energy, right? Most people tell me they don't have enough energy at the end of the day to exercise. Or they say they can't get up early to exercise because they are just too tired. I'm here to let you in on a huge life-changing secret: Working out regularly gives you massive amounts of natural energy!

In addition to regular exercise, here are a couple of other secrets to high energy that I shared with Beth:

- Eating Well
- Being Still
- Giving Back

They are simple, but powerful. These may be new for you,

so hang in there and trust me. Read on:

Eating Well: In addition to the fat loss recommendations I listed earlier, I also shared with Beth other essentials to optimal dietary health:

1. Eat a variety of food colors – e.g., Broccoli, radishes, oranges, apples, blueberries, bananas.
2. Eat rice rather than pasta (unless it's rice pasta)
3. Limit meat consumption

Being Still: If you've never done this, trust me – it works! Your assignment is to quiet yourself for at least a few minutes each morning & night. Sit for 5 – 15 minutes and just focus on your breathing, maybe even focus on one thing you are grateful for. The only rule is *you may not* make a to-do list in your mind. You will be amazed at how calm & focused you will feel once you master this art.

Giving Back: There is nothing more energizing than being of service to another human being. Consider volunteering at your church or local food pantry. Even making an effort to connect with a stranger each day and give them a smile will greatly increase your energy level.

Beth struggled mostly with the 'being still' part of this assignment. I imagine that you will too. Once she got it down, I really noticed a difference in her concentration and her self-esteem.

TO DO: Spend 5 minutes right now, writing down your thoughts and goals for eating well, being still, giving back. If you aren't convinced they work, my challenge to you is to try them for five days. I'd love to hear about your experiences. DrRada@AppleforHealth.com

Secret Revealed

Remember that little secret Beth had been carrying? About 6 weeks into our working together she was finally ready to share. She revealed to me her greatest pain. She also thanked me for holding her accountable for doing her daily quiet time.

It turned out Beth had been engaged about 10 months prior and she was madly in love with her fiancé. But, he continually refused to set a date. When she pressed him further for a reason, he said a horrible thing that left her deeply damaged. He told her he loved her for her mind, but not for her body. Ouch!

Beth took this so deeply to heart that she wouldn't even look at herself in the mirror during training. I didn't get it at first, but now it made perfect sense. In the last 6 week now, she was finally learning she was worth much more than this jerk had to offer and she was now ready to dominate her life:

> **TO DO:** Be fearless when looking at painful past experiences. Everything you've experienced makes you uniquely able to relate to someone – who may be in your shoes now. Embrace your past and help someone who needs you today. You're amazing!

STEP #4:
DOMINATE

This word, especially when applied to a woman, either brings up visions of a dominatrix or a cold-hearted...well you know what. I am here to break another MYTH! Just as men are expected to be the creators of their reality, women are equally equipped to do the same.

As women we have a unique gift of self-awareness. Typically we use this knowledge to hold ourselves back:

- I'm not as good as...
- I'm not as rich as...
- I'm not as skinny as...

You fill in the blanks.

I can promise you when you gain control of your body, you will naturally gain control of your mind. Don't be afraid anymore. You are an amazing person and you just happen to be a woman. It's awesome.

Try these thoughts instead:

- I love how I look...
- I have some amazing ideas...
- I have unique gifts that help others...

You fill in the blanks.

TO DO: If you could wave a magic wand and have any 2 things be true, what would they be? Now work backwards and fill in the "how-to" to accomplish your goals. Truth = you create your reality. You happen to the world. The world does not happen to you anymore.

SUMMARY

Beth reached her goal and has some power-ful wedding photos (remember: her best friend was getting married). She not only regained her physical health, she found her *self* again. It was so great to see her smile!

I dream that all of this can be true for you as well. Stick to these 4 simple steps, use the internet to fill in the blanks, start a weight loss club at work or recruit a trainer to get you there fast! Here's to a bright, beautiful, healthy and vibrant YOU!

I'd like to leave you with these parting thoughts: whatever you want, you can have. But you have to do more than think about it. You have to take action and get help to stay on the right path. All dreams are attainable. I believe in you. Now you must start believing in yourself.

1. Fat Loss
2. Toned & Beautiful Muscles
3. Energized
4. Dominate

If you want to find out more or contact me personally, I can be reached at DrRada@AppleforHealth.com. I am happy to be of service.

Dr. Jennifer Rada DC

ABOUT JENNIFER

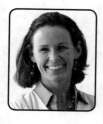

Dr. Jennifer Rada is a Doctor of Chiropractic, a private fitness coach and the author of two life-changing books; *72 Seconds to Success* and *The Fitness Solution*. For over fifteen years, Dr. Jennifer has helped people lose from 10 – 100 pounds and has also worked with specialty groups including: mixed martial artists, wrestlers and bodybuilders.

In her chapter, Dr. Jennifer shows you how to:

- Set goals and get accountable, so you can have the body you've always envisioned!

- Beat the treadmill boredom, so that you can stick to a fitness program that fits your lifestyle, and gets you the results you want!

- Break through frustrating fat loss and muscle-building plateaus, so that you can have more energy, look better and feel better now!

If you're interested in exercise solutions that actually work in the real world, then you're in the right place. Be prepared to breakthrough and breakout to your best body ever!

Dr. Rada's extensive knowledge of anatomy and physiology, combined with her advanced medical training and personal experience in the fitness industry, make her a highly sought after **author, speaker and health coach.**

You can find out more about Dr. Jennifer Rada's services, contact her or request to book her at your next event through her website at: **www.DoctorRada.com**

CHAPTER 14

THE SERENITY SQUEEZE: TURN A LITTLE MUSCLE INTO A GREAT MOVEMENT

BY GEORGE W. CHILDS,
AUTHOR OF *SUCCESSFUL SALES WITHOUT SELLING YOUR SOUL*

Do this exercise first!

Why am I telling you to start here?

If you had discovered a simple new exercise that transformed your life, wouldn't you recommend doing it first?

Have you ever felt that you lacked the motivation to exercise?

Have you ever been so down that you didn't want to get up?

Do you want to know why this doesn't happen to me anymore?

Please do yourself the favor of reading this chapter to the end. You'll learn how to start practicing this new exercise right away. There are so many great exercises in this book. And they'll take you from "flab to fab" so fast it'll make your head spin. But none of these exercises will work for you if you're not motivated to do them.

When you learn how, you'll want to practice the Serenity Squeeze every day. And the best part is... you can do this exercise anywhere, even in bed! In fact, this exercise is likely to help you when you're in bed for other reasons too.

First, let me tell you how I discovered that a little muscle could change my life. As a kid, I was always fidgety. I was so fidgety, I could even wiggle my ears. People often laughed when I wiggled my ears. My Dad made fun of my ears sticking out by saying that I looked like a taxicab with the doors open. My brother would chime in and laugh. I just blushed with embarrassment and somehow failed to notice that their ears stuck out too. My Dad liked to make funny movements with the often overlooked little muscles that we all have.

With a little effort, I learned that I could wiggle my nose at the same time that I wiggled my ears.

Not long thereafter, though, my father died. And I stopped thinking about the funny movements of my little muscles. My ego would like me to say that my father's death was not the defining moment of my life, but I was only 8 years old at the time. My father's death took the wind out of my life's sails. I was always terrified that people would find out that there was something wrong with me. I also feared being perceived as a slacker.

And yet, I was achieving my goals, and doing well in school. When more bad things happened to me (like when my bike got stolen), I got down on myself. I looked for a switch that I could flip or one change that I could make that would get me out of my funk. What I didn't realize was that I had crossed over into being an addict.

I've never taken an illegal drug or misused a prescription drug in my life. I was raised on "Just Say No!" But when I hear a fellow addict talk about drinking something or using a substance because he or she wants to stop feeling so lousy, that's how I felt much of the time. And the hits kept coming.

I was robbed at gunpoint during a home invasion at the age of 24. I had experienced traumatic events before, including a few muggings. But those traumas paled in comparison to a thug threatening to kill me with a gun pointed right at the back of my head.

And as I sat in my bathtub, tied up by the robber, I could feel that this was another turning point in my life ...and one not for the better. To make it through this ordeal, I had to keep thinking straight. The adrenalin was pulsing through my brain so hard that I could barely keep up with the thoughts and fears racing through my mind. I was just trying to survive.

Feeling some neurons in my brain getting fried, I tried to be calm enough to find a way out. I managed to free myself and dialed 9-1-1, escaping any physical injury. I knew I would pay a price for frying my neurons. Ultimately, the price was the hardening of my addiction. At that moment, however, I had no idea how much of my life's time and energy it would cost me.

When PTSD hit me during the months and years that followed, it robbed me of motivation. I became the slacker I had always feared. I was desperate to find that one switch that could make me feel better. Please, let me be clear about one thing. If I were not in recovery for my addictive behaviors in a 12 step program, I would not even have accepted the notion that I deserved the gift of the Serenity Squeeze. Worse still, I would have denied myself its benefits.

Without recovery, I would not be sharing it with you now; I would have nothing to share. Ask me how I found the powerful switch I was looking for, and I will tell you that the Serenity Squeeze found me. In 12 step groups, we talk about a power greater than ourselves restoring us to sanity. The Serenity Squeeze is a gift from my higher power.

I was looking for a way to start exercising again. I wanted a jump-start, some kind of spark that would help me move forward, toward achieving my goals again. What I found was the motivation for a whole new life. I knew that my higher power wanted me to be happy. I experienced joy. I found serenity in a pump, and all I had to do was squeeze it!

How did I prime my Serenity Pump? I started out practicing a breathing technique that Matt Furey taught me at one of his seminars. Although I had heard about breathing being the key to living well, it wasn't until Matt emphasized it that I took it seriously enough to practice it.

Learning to sing in grade school, I was taught to allow my diaphragm to lower while my mid-section expanded, and then to use my abdominal muscles to support the air as it passed over the vocal chords and out my throat. We breathe just like an accordion.

When I read Zen in the Art of Archery, I learned how perplexed Eugen Herrigel became after his Sensei finally told him that pulling the bow was all in the breathing. Why hadn't he mentioned this before? The Sensei explained that had he told him before, Eugen might have thought that learning archery was easy.

Thankfully, Matt Furey, Zen Master of the Internet, didn't wait years to tell me how important breathing is to exercise. And as Matt will tell you, it's not just about breathing, it's also what you do with each breath that counts. Adding a physical movement to each breath, especially on exhale, generates strength. In one of Matt's videos, I learned that pulling up on the anal sphincter while exhaling can build inner strength. "Hmm, a little muscle", I thought, "I can do that."

So, the Serenity Squeeze starts with the following steps:

1. Breathe in through the nose while lowering the diaphragm and extending the navel.

2. Exhale through the nose by pulling the abdominal muscles inward, while simultaneously pulling up on the little muscle surrounding the anal sphincter.

If this sounds like a lot to coordinate, believe me it's not. Once you practice it a few times, you can do this every time you breathe.

I breathe about 10 times a minute when I'm resting, so this means I can practice 50 times in just five minutes. That's 300 times in an hour. If it takes 10,000 practice moves to become an expert, you can become an expert at the Serenity Squeeze in less than a week. What I discovered, however, was that you don't even have to be an expert in order to feel the amazing benefits of this exercise.

And the Serenity Squeeze doesn't end there. If that's all there was to it, I wouldn't be writing this chapter today. One weekend I was in New York City with my wife. While she was at a conference all day, I spent the day as a tourist, walking and taking the subway around the city. I decided to practice my new breathing and squeezing exercise the whole day, not that anyone could tell.

As I continued to practice breathing and squeezing, I noticed that I could also squeeze up on the urogenital diaphragm:

Continue exhaling, while lifting up the perineum right behind the genital area.

The feeling of well-being from squeezing up on this little muscle was amazing! I tried to pull up again on my perineum a little more this time and the pleasurable sensation rose up through my mid-section. After a few more squeezes, I could feel the wave welling up through my core.

Feel the sensation of serenity rising up through your body, to energize the rest of your day.

By the time we flew back home the next day, I was basking in a serene glow of harmonic energy.

Suddenly, my Serenity Pump was primed and I could breathe and squeeze this feeling of serenity anywhere, at anytime. One of the biggest problems that addicts of any kind face is the fear that we can never enjoy life again. With the Serenity Squeeze pumping positive feelings throughout my body, feeling good about myself and my life has banished that fear.

As you practice, keep in mind what I learned as I became a Serenity Squeeze expert:

Void your bladder and your bowels before practicing. You'll be more comfortable and you'll more easily feel the little muscles at work.

When you first learn to practice the Serenity Squeeze, it will be easiest when you are lying in bed. Practice when you wake up for five minutes, and set your reminders for the day. Find quiet time when you won't be interrupted. You want to concentrate on the little muscles.

If you want to practice while sitting, sit on the edge of the seat with your feet planted firmly on the floor. Your posture needs to be "proper" and your breathing relaxed. "Proper" means that your shoulders are pulled back as far as they'll go and your head is up. If you practice while sitting at your desk in front of your computer while you work, you will be pumping serenely in no time.

When you practice the Serenity Squeeze while standing or walking (and breathing correctly), make sure again that your posture is "proper".

Relax and enjoy the exercise. It won't take long to prime your Serenity Pump. Put reminders where you will see them (at your desk, or in your scheduler on your phone) so that you'll remember to practice throughout your day. When you've begun practicing the Serenity Squeeze, don't forget to send me an email to tell me about your experience: George@GeorgeWChilds.com.

As my expertise with the Serenity Squeeze has matured, I can now pull up the urogenital diaphragm in my perineum without engaging the anal sphincter much at all.

When your Serenity Pump starts vibrating like the anti-lock brakes on your car, you'll feel as though you've reached Nirvana.

Enjoy every moment.

One final note: if you've ever done a kegel, it's not the same as the Serenity Squeeze. A kegel is in the same physical neighborhood, but kegels are often done while urinating, or even with an erection if you're male. You pull back to cut off the flow of urine. The Serenity Pump is activated by squeezing up, not back towards the anal sphincter.

If you're ready to build your muscles, so they can burn off your fat, start out with a couple of little muscles. Whether you learn to wiggle your ears or not, the Serenity Squeeze will help build the muscle and reduce the fat between your ears.

You'll be glad you did.

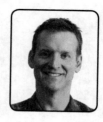

ABOUT GEORGE

George W. Childs grew up in Pittsburgh, PA when the fire from the steel mills still matched the city's passion for its football team. At Tufts University, he met his wife Miya and graduated *Summa Cum Laude*. George started his research career at the Federal Reserve Bank of New York, and trained as an economist at the University of Pennsylvania.

He researched health care services for UPMC until 2002 when he became an entrepreneur for the first time. George grew his retail dry cleaning business to over 30 employees by focusing on serving his customers needs.

Today, George is The Guilt Free Sales Success Mentor, author of *Successful Sales Without Selling Your Soul*, a consultant for buyers and sellers of small businesses, an angel investor, and a mentor to anyone who believes deep down that you can succeed in sales without the fear that you are selling your soul.

George & Miya reside in Pittsburgh with their two children and a pet fish named Steve.

CHAPTER 15

THE SECRET TO LOSING A LARGE AMOUNT OF WEIGHT

BY PAUL REDDICK

I was fat. I couldn't deny it anymore.

This was an embarrassing situation.

Here's why.

Not only was I a certified personal trainer, I worked out too. I ran 30-40 minutes per day.

I thought I was immune to weight gain. I was wrong. The tricky thing about gaining weight is that is "it don't happen overnight." I didn't go to bed one night with a healthy body then wake up the next morning fifty pounds heavier. It happened gradually, a pound here, four or five pounds in a month, then after six months, I'd put on fifty pounds.

Making my living in the baseball world, I'm in front of athletes all the time. I spoke at clinics and camp. I wear a baseball uniform as part of a professional image. Well that uniform was my first real clue that the blubber had started to take over.

It had been over six months since I had to wear a uniform, and when I went to button the pants – the buttons were screaming. The uniform was super tight and the muffin top that overflowed my waistband was extremely uncomfortable. Not a good look.

My solution? I bought a larger size uniform. Problem solved. I was in complete denial that I'd gained weight. I rationalized that the snug fit was due to the uniform shrinking. Even though I knew that I'd gained weight, at this point I was not ready to believe it. I would suck in my stomach...look in the mirror at different angle.... and blame lighting or what I was wearing. The big slap in the face that I'd put on a few pounds was at the mall with my wife. I'd walked past a store window and saw my reflection. I was startled by what I saw; my face was round and my belly protruded over the top of my pants. Ugggh! My initial thought was - I'm fat. Then the rational part of my mind kicked in, "It's a glass reflection, distorted and blurred; and magnified - you're not that fat." I planted this episode at the mall in the back of my mind, but I still would not face the fact that I was fat; denial still had its hold on me. At this point maybe it was delusion.

But, my day of reckoning came when I looked at a set of pictures from a recent vacation. There were too many of them to ignore the reality when I looked at myself. My poses of subconsciously trying to appear thin did not work any longer. Photo after photo showed a person that was no longer in athletic and healthy condition. I was fat. Real fat. This was a rude awakening for me. I am in an industry where looking fit and healthily is a big deal. I felt like Zach Even-Esh.

I was embarrassed and ashamed that I'd let myself get into this shape. I'm a coach, I led a very active lifestyle, I trained pitchers, and I was completely ingrained in the athletic world. But, somehow I let this all slip away.

What is interesting about this point of time in my life was that while this was the fattest I'd ever been, I was still very active. I was running thirty to forty minutes per day and I worked out with the pitchers I was training. With this level of activity I had been able to maintain my physique until my lifestyle changed.

Anyone who works in baseball knows that in order to survive financially, you gain your income from several sources. My workload and my stress level were impacted tremendously. I'd been working for a pro team, doing lessons, teaching part time and writing a lot of books. I also took on a lot of smaller, yet time-consuming projects that were offered to me. With this added workload, my energy level took a nose-dive and my stress level grew. I was still able to workout with my team and I still maintained my running schedule, but even with my aerobic workout instead of maintaining my health…. I was gaining weight.

During this time my diet changed drastically. I was pounding down eighty ounces of coffee per day, which became my sig-nature look, my logo. Eighty ounces of coffee is four large Starbucks mugs. My logic was that drinking more coffee would keep me energized. This did not work. The parents of the kids that I coached would bring me coffee from Dunkin Doughnuts as a thoughtful gesture knowing that I drank a ton of coffee. At the end of the season, the kids even went so far as to commission an artist rendition of me to present as a gift; the drawing illustrated a fat coach – with coffee in hand. Jeez! That was slightly embarrassing.

The coffee and the added cardio workout still did not increase my energy level nor did it influence weight loss. I formed my own theory on what was going on with my body. I'd come to the conclusion that my body had shut down; it no longer considered food as a source of fuel. My body was functioning on a toxic, acidic level. This was because my eating habits had become one of grabbing fast food, gobbling up whatever was convenient and readily available. I was skipping meals, not eating enough to maintain a healthy metabolism. I'd delay eating until I came home. I ate too much... too late at night. With the added stress in my life, I'm certain my hormone levels were out of balance, which heavily factored in prevented me from losing weight and factored into my decrease in energy.

I became desperate on what to do. While I'd come to terms with accepting that I'd gained a lot of weight, I'd yet to come to terms with doing anything about it – that is, until I revisited my vacation photos. The man in those photos was not the man I wanted to be. I knew something had to be different; I could not live like this any longer.

I had to go back to the drawing board and come up with a new plan for a new lifestyle, ... a plan that would work. I began following a high intensity interval training program developed by a buddy of mine, Mike Shele. He owns The Training Room in Avon, New Jersey. The interval program was based on Mike's body weight exercises. I wanted to workout out at home so I did not want equipment to hold me back. So, bodyweight was perfect. I did use a kettlebell, but that was the only weight I used.

Following Mike's plan I mixed up the intervals.... they were forty seconds-on, forty seconds-off, twenty seconds-on, twenty seconds-off, thirty seconds-on, thirty seconds-off and so on.

I followed Mike's program via a website and I did all the training in my living room.

This high intensity interval training cut my workout sessions in half. I had been running forty minutes per day plus the time it took me to stretch would add up to approximately sixty minutes per day.

The interval training ran a little more than twenty minutes per day. As a result of these high intensity interval training sessions I shed thirty to forty pounds relatively quickly. I accomplished this weight loss just by using the interval training protocol only. I was not using any other training program.

During this time, I ran into a fitness and diet expert, Jeff Cavaliere. I confided in him that I lost forty pounds and I was now dedicated to getting healthier as well as getting my body into shape. He put me on his eating plan, but the great thing about this diet was that it was implemented in stages – no radical transformations.

The first week he did not have me do anything different with my choice of foods, he had me increase my food intake. He told to eat a meal every two and a half to three hours. This was easily accomplished as my eating habits had improved a little bit, but they were still out of control. The awesome result from this new eating regime was I still continued to lose weight even though I was eating more food on a daily basis.

The next week, Jeff introduced me to protein shakes and bars with which I replaced some of the bad foods I had been eating. These worked great. Between meals I would have either a protein shake or a bar. I liked this because I knew exactly what I was putting into my body; they took out the guesswork. Instead of me eating a salad with hidden fat and packing in two thousand calories of salad dressing that I was unaware of, I was able to control the content of my food intake.

With this diet plan, I was able to lose the final ten to fifteen pounds. I went from weighing two hundred and fifty pounds to my lowest weight of one hundred and ninety. I continue with the high intensity interval training; I've actually moved closer to Mike's gym and attend his group classes every week. My weight fluctuates between 195 to 205lbs.

But, the most important transformation is that I feel great, and I like the way I look. I have no issues with my eating and I am able to maintain the program. I do have cheat days when I fall off the wagon and eat the wrong foods from time to time, but I am able get right back on it because the program is so easy to follow.

I also learned to manage my workload better. By streamlining my time management my stress level went way down. As a result, my coffee intake dropped sixty percent. I still love my coffee… but, I now drink approximately sixteen ounces of coffee in the morning and twelve ounces around noon. The other simple changes I've added to my weight maintenance program are that I've added the proper supplements. I now take a multivitamin, fish oil, fiber supplement and calcium. I drink a liter of water in the morning and a liter of water before I go to bed to stay hydrated.

I got rid of all those bad carbs too. I've eliminated all the white carbohydrates from my diet, foods such as potatoes, pasta, rice and white bread. I've added more whole grain carbohydrates or what Jeff has termed fibrous carbs. Foods such as shakes that are strategically-engineered for optimum carbohydrate recovery, sprouted grain bread, and fibrous whole grain couscous. I consciously avoid all the starchy carbohydrates that spiked my blood sugar and influenced my insulin levels.

There was a combination of factors that contributed to my weight loss. I reduced my stress levels tremendously by managing my workload more efficiently. I continued my high intensity interval training using body weight and kettle-bells. I was no longer involved in that cardio madness where more does not mean better.

It was not difficult to cut my workout routine in half. A twenty-minute workout can easily fit into a daily schedule. Jeff's meal plans were easy to incorporate and it didn't make eating for me a punishment or monotonous.

The results from the 'before' and 'after' photos speak for themselves. It has been an unbelievable transformation. I look great, I feel great simply by altering my exercise program, reducing stress levels, getting my diet under control, and gaining control of my work schedule. The result is I lost fifty pounds.

It's easy to get off track and lose focus. I was locked into bad habits that I formed over many months. All the areas of my life were out of control. The amazing part of making these lifestyle changes was that I didn't pressure myself to modify all the areas of my life at once. I implemented them in stages – this approach was a seamless progression that worked for me.

My advice to anyone wanting to lose weight and become healthier is to start slowly, realize that you did not get into the shape you are in overnight, and you won't get out of it overnight. These adjustments require very little willpower and all you need to do is believe that you can turn it around.

Best of luck to you.

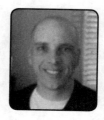

ABOUT PAUL

Paul Reddick helps pitchers throw harder. Because of the results of the pitchers that use his many books, courses and instruction, Paul is known as the Master Of MPH. Paul has served as a scout for the Pittsburgh Pirates, a state delegate for USA Baseball and coached in the Montreal Expo farm system.

His signature velocity-getting course *The 90mph Club* is used by more pitchers than any other single pitching training program.

Paul is currently the Director of The Yogi Berra Museum baseball camp and the Co-Author of the best seller *The Picture Perfect Pitcher* with Tom House and Mike Epstein on *Hitting with Mike Epstein*.

He's been featured in Collegiate Baseball News, Baseball America, Junior Baseball Magazine, NBC News, News 12, The Newark Star Ledger, and starred in the T.V. pilot *The 25th Man*.

In 2010,Newark Mayor Cory Booker presented Paul with The Larry Doby award for service to the youth of Newark.

Paul is also one of America's top young speakers. He speaks to numerous youth, high school, college, and business groups every year. Paul's speaking career is centered around empowering youth and college groups to achieve lasting success, greater friendships, and healthy relationships.

Baseball legend Yogi Berra say's "Paul's a great coach. He really knows his stuff."

CHAPTER 16

THE MIRACLE WAY TO BURN FAT FAST!

BY MATT FUREY

I f you haven't watched the movie *Miracle* yet, I suggest you get a copy of the DVD and make it top-shelf viewing, for yourself and anyone close to you. Since my first viewing of the movie about the 1980 U.S.A. Olympic Hockey team's victory over the Soviet's, I've repeatedly tuned into a segment from it that you can truly relate to, especially if you've been following my program, *The Fastest Way Humanly Possible to Burn Fat.*

The segment I'm referring to is when head coach Herb Brooks had the team skating wind sprints immediately after an unenthusiastic game against the Norwegians. During the game the athletes were staring off into the stands, pointing out the "hot" women seated in various sections. Coach Brooks silently cringed and took note of the team's lack of focus, and corrected it by nearly running them to death.

As I watched the players doing "red line-blue line" sprints, which they un-affectionately referred to as "Herbies" I yearned to learn more about how they trained.

When you sit and watch the entire movie (it's 2.5 hours long), you'll probably be amazed at how fast the action moves. Talk about time-distortion. The entire movie feels like 15 minutes, which is the sign of something truly epic.

I watched it with my son and it gave both of us a megadose of motivation to get more done, to accomplish more goals, to reach for the stars and hit them.

One of the most important lines in the movie *Miracle*, is hurled across the ice when the men are doing sprints at the end of practice. As they burst across the ice on their skates, Coach Brooks tells everyone they better get used to this drill as they'll be doing it a lot.

A bit later he hollers, *"The legs feed the wolf."* When I heard this line I hit the rewind button and played it again and again. Then I took out a pen and wrote it in my journal.

GREAT COACHES ARE OBSESSED WITH CONDITIONING

A couple days later, I was still thinking about the phrase and its meaning. Like coaches I have had throughout my career, including Dan Gable and Karl Gotch, Herb Brooks was ob-sessed with conditioning. To him, "the legs feed the wolf" meant that great hockey players, like wolves on the hunt, need a combination of speed and endurance.

Karl Gotch referred to conditioning as "your best hold." He didn't emphasize speed as much as strength-endurance, as speed came from having good timing and reflexes.

Dan Gable was fanatical about conditioning as well. At the University of Iowa he often had us doing sprints around the top floor of the arena – a good ¼ mile, if I'm calculating correctly. He also had us do sprints at the end of practice in the wrestling room as well as up the arena steps. Some of these uphill sprints including carrying another on your back, hence the name "buddy carries."

At Edinboro, the year I won the NCAA II title, Bruce Baumgartner, a 2-time Olympic Gold Medalist and 4-time Olympic medalist at heavyweight, had us mix sprints with calisthenics like pushups, v-ups and pull-ups. On my own, I did them on a stationary cycle after warming up in the sauna.

The following season, for whatever reason, our coaches sprinted us less often, and I did so far less often myself. Because hindsight is often perfect, I can tell you this was a mistake and if I had the year to do over, I'd have run the sprints – and pedaled them, too.

"THE LEGS FEED THE WILL."

I have a couple other ways of explaining the benefits of *"the legs feed the wolf."* One is that sprints or speed-endurance work triggers your body to release more *yang* energy. When you sprint, you not only get faster and generate more endurance – you also turn back the clock and cause your body to get younger.

Sprinting also causes your body to naturally secrete more HGH and testosterone, whereas long-distance cardio causes the opposite reaction.

Another way I look at *"the legs feed the wolf"* involves a slight word variation. By changing the word 'wolf' to 'will' we have even more meaning.

"The legs feed the *will*."

What does this mean?

Well, when you sprint you cause the lungs, the kidneys and the heart to get stronger. They either adapt – or else. And when the organs of the body are strengthened, so are the muscles.

If someone is weak-willed, his kidneys are weak. If he is strong-willed, his kidneys serve him well. One of my favorite Chinese sayings is, *"Ren lao, xian lao tui."* This means, when a person gets old, his legs go first.

Strong legs not only feed the wolf, they also feed the will. It takes a strong will and great determination to run sprint after sprint when your lungs are gasping for air. It takes guts or that quality we call "intestinal fortitude" to muster the mental and physical energy to make your fast and super-fast twitch muscle fibers fire on command.

Putting collegiate, Olympic or professional athletes on a sprinting program is fairly easy. Most are relatively young and their bodies are durable. Even if they don't fully recover from one workout to the next, they can usually get by without the risk of injury.

START SPRINTING...SLOWLY

But most people must start out slowly with sprints – and build up over several months. It would be utter foolishness to attempt sprint after sprint, day after day, if your body isn't used to it – even if it seemed like no big deal if you used to do them years ago and think you know what you're doing. You might – but does your body know what you're doing?

Even when you start out with 30-40 percent sprints – your

body begins to adapt very quickly. Your metabolism receives the message: Burn fat – FAST. Your central nervous system gets the message: grow younger. And your brain gets sharper, including a better memory and a keener sense of what is going on around you.

In addition to the above, with sprints you can count on other benefits other than burning fat. Expect cholesterol levels, triglyceride levels and blood sugar levels to get healthier and stabilize.

Oh, and about that other urge – you can expect to see a jump there as well. Why? Because when you sprint, you not only engage the kidneys – but the by-product of strong kidneys is strong sexual function. Not only that, but provided you're hitting the balls of your feet when you sprint (not your heels), those of you who are men will discover that your other "balls" start working better, too.

Yes, I've started many people out with a handful of bursts done at 30 to 40% of their perceived maximum. And they were absolutely stunned at how sprints at less than "full bore" could still yield superior results to anything they've ever tried before.

THE FASTEST WAY TO BURN FAT ON A BASEBALL DIAMOND

Now, you might be thinking, I don't have any hills, or a hockey rink, or a nice grassy meadow to run sprints. If so, let me open your mind to all the other places where you can sprint yourself into fantastic physical condition.

In football you'll hear the equivalent of "Herbies" being called "gassers." In basketball, they're "suicides." In wrestling we called them "rat races."

THE DEFINITIVE GUIDE TO BURNING FAT AND BUILDING MUSCLE

And now, because of my involvement in the sport of baseball, I like to call them Fure-cats. Why? Because I've never seen them done in baseball the way I teach.

How to do them?

Well, if you're all alone, the answer is easy. So let me cover that first, followed by how to run an entire group through them.

SOLO FURE-CATS

To do Fure-cats by yourself, all you need is a baseball diamond. A Little League field is fine, regardless of whether or not it's used for baseball or softball. The size of the diamond is also irrelevant. You can make it work on any field from the MLB to t-ball, indoor or outdoor.

Instructions for Solo Fure-cats:

1. Run around the diamond, from home plate to first, to second, to third and back to home, for about 3-5 minutes to warm-up. This warm-up is NOT a sprint. It's a light run. Nothing more.
2. After your warm-up, do 5-10 minutes of joint loosening exercises, as seen in *Combat Stretching*.
3. After the joint loosening exercises, walk between first and second base. While doing so, put down two markers. Doing so will give you four markers in total because first and second base are also markers. Make sure all four markers are evenly divided.
4. Markers can be as simple as a line you draw in the dirt with your foot, or a stick or cone.
5. Once all your markers are evenly distributed, put one foot on first base with the other leading toward second.
6. Get mentally ready by telling yourself that this first

Fure-cat will be run at 40% of your maximum.

7. At 40%, sprint to the first marker and immediately pivot and sprint back to first. Immediately turn again and sprint to the second marker. Turn again and sprint to first. As soon as you touch first, turn again and sprint all the way to second base. And as soon as you touch second, turn and sprint all the way back to first base. This completes your first sprint.

8. When you finish this first sprint, do NOT sit down. Do NOT stand around. To recover, walk around slowly with your hands behind your head. Expand your lungs. Breathe deeply. Continue walking slowly for 90 seconds to 2 minutes. By then you will most likely be fully recovered.

9. Take a small drink of water – then get on the line for sprint #2.

10. Do sprint #2 the same as #1, at 40%.

11. Recover the same way, by walking around slowly and taking a small sip of water.

12. Do the next sprint at 40-50% of your maximum.

13. Recover the same way as before.

14. Do the fourth sprint at 50-60% of your maximum.

15. Recover the same as before.

16. Assess where you are at this point. You may be done for the day. If this is your first time doing a sprint like this, I recommend only doing four. If you've been doing hill sprints and such, as taught in *The Fastest Way Humanly Possible to Burn Fat*, then you can do more. Just keep in mind that this type of sprinting, because of the quick stops and turns, works even more fast twitch and super-fast twitch muscle fibers than the other types of sprints. This type of sprint will also get you even more

winded than a regular burst.

17. When you've completed all your Fure-cats – walk around slowly for several minutes to recover. Drink plenty of water (not the sports drinks that are loaded with sugars).

18. Eat a protein meal after this workout – but avoid any type of sugar for at least one full hour – but preferably at least two. This will ensure that your body releases a mega-dose of HGH – the hormone that keeps you younger, stronger and healthier.

3 PERSON FURE-CATS

If you're doing Fure-cats as a group of three, you can take turns. When one guy is sprinting, someone is timing him and giving encouragement. When the first person is finished and recovering, the second person is sprinting and the third person is acting as coach.

12 PERSON GROUP

In Little League, it's typical to have 11 or 12 kids on the squad. So here's what I do: I have six boys go to first base and the other six go to third base.

Then I make two marks between each base. Group A will sprint back and forth between first and second base. Group B will sprint back and forth between third and second base. No one in either group will ever cross second base. This is very important to avoid collisions of any sort.

When I blow the whistle, both groups run at the same time. Both groups recover by walking around slowly. Drink plenty of water. Line both groups up and repeat till satisfied.

TRACK YOUR PROGRESS

If you really like Fure-cats and want to make them a regular feature of your sprint training, keep in mind that this workout is not done everyday. Two or three times per week is ideal.

I encourage you to keep a log on when you sprinted. Answer the following questions in your log:

What day did I sprint?

What time of day did I sprint?

What percentage of my maximum did I give for each sprint?

What were my times?

For the warm-up sprints, you may not want to time yourself because the clock does seem to compel some people to run faster before it is ideal. If you can control yourself, then you can time each and every sprint.

FOCUS ON BURNING FAT, NOT ON LOSING WEIGHT

As you sprint and track your progress, you're far better off looking at and analyzing how much fat you burned. Remember this: The scale doesn't tell you whether you lost fat, water or muscle – yet far too many people rely on it as if it's the only true measure of fitness.

You'll do much better and stay motivated if you put far less emphasis on the scale and more upon how you look and feel. Photographic proof is fantastic. So is looking at how you fit into your clothes. And it's hard to go wrong with a simple body fat test.

Focus your mind on burning fat and building muscle and a

health and fitness "miracle" will take place as you transform your life.

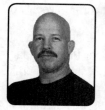

ABOUT MATT

Matt Furey was born in a small town in Iowa, named Carroll.

At eight years of age he began competing in swimming and wrestling and through dedicated practice became a champion in both. In 1981, Matt Furey was the state runner-up in the Class 3A Iowa High School State Wrestling Championships at 167-pounds. He attended The University of Iowa from 1981-1984, where he wrestled for Olympic Gold medalist, Dan Gable, and was a member of three national championship teams.

In the fall of 1984, in order to help rebuild a doormat wrestling program, Furey transferred to Edinboro University of Pennsylvania, and in 1985 he won the NCAA II national title at 167-pounds, defeating two-time California state champion, Howard Lawson, in the finals. While at Edinboro he was coached by Mike DeAnna and two-time Olympic Gold Medalist Bruce Baumgartner.

In February of 1987, Furey opened a personal training business for wrestlers and fitness enthusiasts. Most of the high school wrestlers he trained went on to wrestle in college.

Furey began studying various martial arts in 1990 and immediately saw the physical, mental and philosophical links these arts had with wrestling. This lead to the publication of his first book and videos in 1996, entitled, *The Martial Art of Wrestling*.

Also in 1996, Furey began competing in the ancient Chinese grappling art of Shuai-Chiao, the oldest style of kung fu. Furey's teacher, Dr. Daniel Weng, a national champion from Taiwan, and a ninth-degree black belt, guided Furey to three national titles.

During Christmas of 1997, Dr. Weng brought two U.S. teams to Beijing, China, to compete in the world championships. In Beijing, Furey won the gold medal at 90 KG (198-pounds), and was the only non-Chinese to win a title. In addition, Furey's world title was historic because it marked the first time that an American had won a gold medal in any world kung fu competition held in China.

In the spring of 1998, Furey was inducted into the Edinboro University of Pennslyvania Athletic Hall of Fame.

In 1999, Furey traveled to Tampa, Florida to train under the legendary Karl Gotch. Several months later Furey moved his family from California to Tampa, Florida, so he could train with Gotch full-time. Gotch taught Furey a treasure trove of knowledge on conditioning as well as the real professional style of wrestling, known as catch-as-catch-can (catch wrestling).

Furey's unique experience as a Chinese kung fu and wrestling champion, earned him covers for *Grappling, Inside Kung Fu, Karate Illustrated, Gladiator* and *Martial Arts Illustrated*.

In 2002, *Grappling* magazine dubbed Furey, "The King of Catch Wrestling" – and in the book *Grappling Masters*, Furey is one of 22 elite world class grapplers who are interviewed and featured.

In 2010, *Inside Kung Fu* named Furey as their *Hall of Fame Writer of the Year*.

Furey is also the author of the international best-selling **Combat Conditioning**, as well as **Combat Abs**, *The Unbeatable Man, 101 Ways to Magnetize Money, The Fastest Way Humanly Possible to Burn Fat*, **Combat Stretching**, **Gama Fitness** and **Magnetic Mind Power**.

As President of *The Psycho-Cybernetics Foundation*, Furey is dedicated to spreading the teachings of Dr. Maxwell Maltz, author of the 30-million copy best-seller, *Psycho-Cybernetics*.

Along with his wife and two children, Furey resides in Tampa, Florida and Hainan Island, China.